Bodybuilding, Drugs and Risk

Current popular interest in bodies, fitness, sport and active lifestyles, has made bodybuilding more visible and acceptable within mainstream society than ever before. However, the association between bodybuilding, drugs and risk has contributed to a negative image of an activity which many people find puzzling.

Using data obtained from participant observation and interviews, this book explores bodybuilding subculture from the bodybuilders' perspectives. It looks at:

- how bodybuilders try to maintain competent social identities
- how they manage the risks of using steroids and other physique-enhancing drugs
- how they understand the alleged steroid-violence link
- how they 'see' the muscular body

Through systematic exploration it becomes apparent that previous attempts to explain bodybuilding in terms of a 'masculinity-in-crisis' or gender insecurity are open to question. Difficult questions about what sustains and legitimates potentially dangerous bodily practices are provided by this detailed picture of a huge underground subculture.

Lee F. Monaghan is lecturer in Sociology at the Cardiff School of Social Sciences, Cardiff University.

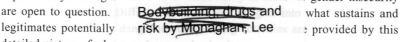

HEALTH, RISK AND SOCIETY

Series editor
Graham Hart
MRC Social and Public Health Sciences Unit, Glasgow

In recent years, social scientific interest in risk has increased enormously. In the health field, risk is seen as having the potential to bridge the gap between individuals, communities and the larger social structure, with a theoretical framework which unifies concerns around a number of contemporary health issues. This new series will explore the concept of risk in detail, and address some of the most active areas of current health and research practice.

Previous title in this series:

Risk and misfortune
Judith Green

The endangered self: managing the social risk of HIV
Gill Green and Elisa J. Sobo

Bodybuilding, Drugs and Risk

Lee F. Monaghan

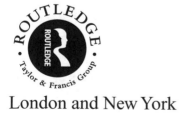

London and New York

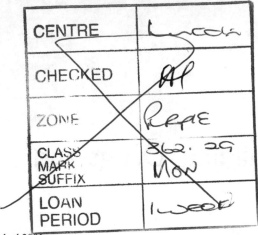

First published 2001
by Routledge
11 New Fetter Lane, London EC4P 4EE

Simultaneously published in the USA and Canada
by Routledge
29 West 35th Street, New York, NY 10001

Routledge is an imprint of the Taylor & Francis Group

© 2001 Lee F. Monaghan

Typeset in Times by
HWA Text and Data Management, Tunbridge Wells
Printed and bound in Great Britain by
TJ International Ltd, Padstow, Cornwall

British Library Cataloguing in Publication Data
A catalogue record for this book is available from the British
Library

Library of Congress Cataloging in Publication Data
Monaghan, Lee F., 1972–
    Bodybuilding, drugs and risk / Lee F. Monaghan.
        p. cm. – (Health, risk and society)
    Includes bibliographical references and index.
        1. Doping in sports. 2. Bodybuilders–Drug use.
    3. Anabolic steroids. I. Title. II. Series.

RC1230 .M65 2001
362.29′088′796–dc21   00–062722

ISBN 0-415-22682-1 (hbk)
ISBN 0-415-22683-X (pbk)

To Beccie and Niamh

Contents

Tables

Preface

Experts, and expert systems of knowledge, have a particular place in the 'risk society'. They contribute to the production of risk, to risk measurement and to its management. Access to experts, and expert systems, however limited, allows us to more clearly refine the nature of exposure to health risks, and to minimise the harms associated with production, consumption and everyday life. Expert control over knowledge has always been challenged, via the 'underground' printing and reproduction of texts, but a major change to have occurred in recent years is the extent to which expert knowledge that was previously difficult to acquire, or contained within highly regulated professional boundaries and spaces, has become available to a much wider audience. The current revolution in information and communications technology – in particular, through the internet – allows unprecedented access to highly technical information, as well as to groups and individuals who are willing to interpret, question, modify and summarise this knowledge.

In *Bodybuilding, Drugs and Risk* Lee Monaghan shows how one group has appropriated a very specific and arcane body of information – on the pharmacology and indeed pharmokinetics of anabolic-androgenic steroids and associated pharmaceutical products – for the purpose of physique enhancement. In medical terms steroid use is a high risk activity: by taking non-prescribed, illicit drugs, bodybuilders risk serious physical side effects and even death. Some would argue that bodybuilders either have, or are at risk of, a psychological disorder – muscle dysmorphia, the physical 'opposite' of *anorexia nervosa*. Yet as Monaghan shows, many of the bodybuilders he contacted had a very sophisticated, highly nuanced and intricate grasp of chemical interactions and the body's response to them, and indeed this corpus of knowledge – entirely outside of formal pharmacopoeia – can be described as a discrete 'ethnopharmacology'.

PREFACE

This is risk management with a difference. The detailed knowledge of body-builders, male and female, allows them to both push their bodies to previously unimaginable limits, whilst maintaining sufficient control so that muscles do not tear apart, livers can still process drugs (at least in the short and medium term) and hearts do not – literally – burst. This is all done in a particular *habitus*: the social world of gyms, among supportive peers with whom to share and compare new information, and partners who validate and are sometimes themselves participants in the milieu. The risks are not exclusively physical or mental. The social risk here is of stigmatisation, being stereotyped as violent and unintelligent ('all brawn and no brain') and, through the production of hypermuscular physiques, of taking beyond what is considered acceptable the (re-)construction and management of the body.

Lee Monaghan describes this world, its inhabitants and structures of knowledge in a way that completely undermines the public representations of bodybuilding, to bring us a picture of men and women who are as thoughtful, reflexive and insightful as any group with a specialised human interest. Their engagement with and expertise in the complex pharmacology of drug use gives us a whole new perspective on risk in society, demonstrating how knowledge cannot be restricted to a single domain or remain the provenance only of credited experts. Bodybuilders' everyday knowledge challenges current limits on access to information and its practical application, and demonstrates its place in confronting, living and working with risk. This contribution to the *Health, Risk and Society* series is most welcome, and takes us further along the road of understanding that knowledge and technologies generated for one purpose, can have other functions and be put to other uses; with scientific advances come new risks, new means of avoiding established risks, and applications with myriad unintended consequences. *Bodybuilding, Drugs and Risk* provides us with a remarkable insight into a previously unseen world of knowledge, risk and expertise.

Graham Hart
Series Editor
Health, Risk and Society

Acknowledgements

In writing this book I have incurred many debts. I would like to thank everybody who contributed, either directly or indirectly, to this work. First and foremost, I wish to express my gratitude to all my ethnographic contacts. In preserving anonymity I will not identify these people by name. One man in particular, whom I call Soccer, was particularly helpful. As well as providing me with many insights he enabled me to tap into a network of drug-using bodybuilders.

This manuscript, edited by Graham Hart to whom I owe my thanks, is based on a doctoral thesis completed in 1997 at Cardiff University. I would like to thank everybody who assisted me during that three-year project. Undoubtedly, my deepest debt is owed to Michael Bloor who acted diligently as my supervisor. Neil McKeganey, who was informative in the writing of the original manuscript, rightly describes Michael Bloor as a sociologists' sociologist. Many thanks also go to Russell and Rebecca Dobash for their academic support and encouragement.

Funds were obtained during the first two years of study from the Economic and Social Research Council (ESRC), for which I am grateful. My last year of funding was provided by the School of Social and Administrative Studies, Cardiff University. (Currently The Cardiff School of Social Sciences.) I wish to thank the School for awarding me departmental funding in order to complete the original thesis. Other current and former colleagues in the School to whom I am indebted include Sara Delamont, Paul Atkinson, Ian Shaw, Samantha Edwards, Jill Bourne, Anna Weaver, Joanna Wilkes, Sharon Bechares, Irene Williams and Liz Renton. Many thanks also go to those who typed interview transcripts, especially Joan Ryan and Caroline Eason. Several clinicians and service agency providers catering for steroid users also helped during the research process. A big thank you is owed to Andrew McBride, Kathyrn Williamson, Dick Pates, Phil Coles, Joe Molloy, Guy Thomas, Colin Ranshaw, Huw Perry and Nick Evans.

ACKNOWLEDGEMENTS

Some of the material in this book has appeared in a slightly different form elsewhere. I am grateful to Mike Featherstone and Sage Publications for permission to reprint material from L. Monaghan (1999) 'Creating "the perfect body": a variable project', *Body & Society* 5, 2–3: 267–90. Similarly, I wish to thank Jonathan Gabe and Blackwell Publishers for permission to reprint material from L. Monaghan (1999) 'Challenging medicine? Bodybuilding, drugs and risk', *Sociology of Health & Illness* 22, 3: 707–34.

My parents, Francis and Maureen Monaghan, deserve my thanks. Their love, support and encouragement over the years is greatly appreciated. Finally, writing this book, while also undertaking other research projects and starting a new lecturing post, inevitably impinged upon family time. For that reason not least, my wife and daughter deserve this book's dedication.

'Many scientists feel we are entering a golden age of drug development. The use of both old and new substances in athletics will grow proportionately. Without doubt it will be an interesting time and a critical one both medically and philosophically' (Wright 1982: 6).

'It is my firm belief that you cannot hold a comprehensive discussion about bodybuilding, or any other sports for that matter, without talking about the use of anabolic steroids and other performance-enhancing drugs' (Phillips 1997a: 42).

Chapter 1

Introduction: risking the physical and social self

The new Millennium, with its promise of new opportunities and technologies, lays witness to recurring 'social problems' including what many consider the scourge of modern sport: drug-taking for athletic enhancement. The clandestine use of biochemical resources in the risk oriented world of late modernity (Beck 1992, Giddens 1991) is one of the few issues which shifts the focus on sport to the front pages of newspapers (Bromley 1997: 112). As sports become increasingly capital intensive, it is unsurprising that some athletes competing in the 2000 Olympic Games have been discredited for taking banned/hazardous drugs such as anabolic-androgenic steroids (hereafter abbreviated to steroids). However, as evidenced in the British press during previous Olympic Games, it is not only elite athletes who risk drug side effects and social stigmatisation. Bodybuilders, in particular, have been negatively characterised as (among other things) illicit steroid 'abusers' (*The Guardian* 6 August 1992). Here risks to the Olympic ethic of 'fair play' are substituted by concerns of self-other health risks, including drug induced violence.

The imposition of risk has a moral dimension (Douglas 1990). While risk may be glorified and its virtues extolled (Adams 1995: 16–17), people voluntarily engaging in behaviours which medicine labels as 'risk-inducing' are typically categorised as 'irresponsible' (Lane 1995: 61). To be sure, bodybuilding and drug-taking are not synonymous, and many bodybuilders are well motivated to resist the vocabulary of risk. Nevertheless, the reported global 'abuse' of steroids among gym members – anomalous with the supposed healthism of exercise and widely considered dangerous and polluting (Douglas 1966) – renders 'bodybuilder' synonymous with the pejorative label 'risk taker' in many people's minds. Within

Western scientific and popular discourse such deviancy is claimed to manifest in the materiality of the body (Shildrick 1998: 113). A possible long-term hazard of drug-assisted bodybuilding, not immediately apparent but instead dependent upon the probing of biomedical science, is damage to internal bodily organs such as the liver, kidneys and cardiovascular system (Kashkin 1992). Moreover, the marking of deviancy on 'excessively' muscular fe/male bodies in a more recognisable fashion – the inscription and projection of powerful cultural meanings – represents another possible risk for those bodybuilders who transgress the normative ideal of the 'fit-looking' body. As stated by St Martin and Gavey (1996: 47):

> It has been suggested that the greatest public discomfort about body-builders is that 'all those muscles somehow come out of a bottle; that there is something as synthetic, unhealthy, useless and faintly sinful as plastic flowers about what they do and the way they look' (Gaines and Butler, 1980: 76); that there is discomfort about 'the impurity of the chemical body, the unnaturalness of the steroid body' (Mansfield and McGinn, 1993: 59).

While those bodybuilders who are also drug users may be risking their health, all bodybuilders risk stigmatisation given 'the way they look' and the 'suspect' nature of their subcultural affiliations. The maligned view that all bodybuilders – irrespective of individual (in)experience with steroids and analogous compounds – are narcissistic, inadequate and socially irresponsible drug 'abusers' is a form of cultural stereotyping which is conceivably threatening to self-identity (Goffman 1968). In such a context risk becomes manifold; possible adverse consequences of being a (drug-taking) bodybuilder relate to the physical and social self.

A necessary condition for individual commitment to this demonised 'drug-abusing' subculture is a different, more positive, definition of bodybuilding activities, muscular bodies and identities. Similar to research on illicit drug-taking conducted in the same vein as anthropological studies of native life (e.g. McKeganey and Barnard 1992), this book provides an ethnographic picture. Using detailed qualitative data largely obtained from South Wales bodybuilders, it explores the sustainability of the 'risky' practice of bodybuilding as participants endeavour to construct and maintain 'appropriate' bodies and identities.

Before reporting and analysing empirical data it is necessary to contextualise the study. After clarifying my use of the terms drug 'users' and 'abusers', the following briefly reviews some relevant literature and provides an overview of the research, study sample and chapter content.

Drug 'users' or 'abusers'?

Bodybuilders self-administering drugs such as steroids 'do not perceive themselves to be drug users in the same way that amphetamine or heroin users are' (Pates and Temple 1992: 5). When a South Wales needle exchange began to provide injecting equipment suitable for steroid users (who, because they normally inject into muscle tissue, require larger needles than intravenous injectors), exchange staff were asked by steroid-using clients if staff would schedule separate sessions for steroid users, as they did not like mixing with the exchange's other 'junkie' clientele.

This self-differentiation, evidenced among other drug-using populations (*cf.* Davis and Munoz 1968), is understandable. The maligned 'drug taker' label is synonymous with 'risk taker' in popular thought. However, 'objectively' speaking, bodybuilders are taking drugs if ingesting or injecting steroids and analogous compounds (e.g. Clenbuterol, Diuretics, Gonadotrophic Stimulants and Human Growth Hormone). Bodybuilders' vocabularies of motive for drug use, specifically, justifications through an appeal to normality (Weinstein 1980: 582), enable users to concede this and retain competent social identity. For example, terms such as 'medicines', 'hormones', 'supplements' and 'pharmaceuticals' may be used instead of 'drug'. Because many bodybuilders accept that their physique-enhancing compounds are 'drugs' – just as alcohol, aspirin, tobacco and caffeine are 'drugs' – the term is used in this study. Similarly, 'use' and the explicitly discriminatory term 'abuse' are employed. The meanings of these terms, which carry connotations of personal characteristics like responsibility and culpability, are clarified below:

For the most part these terms correlate with members' understandings as opposed to culturally dominant definitions of what constitutes proper and improper behaviour. For bodybuilders, the meaning of these terms has little to do with whether substances are prescribed by a clinician, used for their stated medical purpose, or whether moral and legal rules are broken.

According to experienced bodybuilders, generalised and flexible parameters exist for effective experimental investigation of drugs with a minimum risk to health. For example, long-term users claim there are 'correct' ways of taking bodybuilding drugs which entails (among other things) a full knowledge of pharmacological 'chain reactions' (Goldstein 1990: 91). For bodybuilders abuse is equated with overuse, indiscriminate use and unplanned taking with an absence of control. Taking chemicals without correct training and dietary regimens also betokens abusers as opposed to users (Bloor *et al.* 1998). Significantly, all steroid-using bodybuilders contacted during this research claimed they used these drugs correctly, except in a few instances when the responsible narrator admitted to previous abuse as a novice. Persons abusing steroids and analogous drugs are similar to 'junkies' in the bodybuilders' ideational world. According to bodybuilders these third parties are often psychologically (rather than physiologically) addicted to steroids.

As a qualitative study, bodybuilders' understandings are prioritised. In detailing bodybuilding and the instrumental use of various different substances, this book is attentive to 'the social and cultural context in which drug use occurs and, viewing drug use from the point of view of the drug user [aims to] show the meaning drug use has in [the drug users'] lives' (Taylor 1993: 5). Hence, drug-taking in body-building is, for the most part, described as use not abuse. When bodybuilders' drug-taking constitutes improper use (as judged by subcultural criteria), this is described as abuse. When bodybuilders' drug-taking is noted from an 'outsider' stance, abuse is placed in scare quotes ('abuse'). Drug-taking is an expression used interchangeably with drug use and is employed to avoid undue repetition.

The literature

This research extends over several areas which cannot be reviewed exhaustively. This section briefly reviews *some* relevant academic literature on 'reflexive' bodies and identities in risk society, bodybuilding subculture, steroids and violence. Selectivity does not mean other writings are irrelevant. For example, this book contributes to an ongoing tradition of ethnographic research on drug subcultures, providing a corrective to influential cultural theories of risk (Douglas and Calvez 1990) which characterise injecting drug users as 'isolates' (or fatalists) with low group integration (Bloor 1995: 95).

Reflexive bodies and identities in risk society

Contributors to the recently established sociology of the body (e.g. Nettleton and Watson 1998, Shilling 1993), reference Giddens (1991) when contextualising a burgeoning social scientific interest in bodily matters. According to Giddens, contemporary society (what he terms 'high' or 'late' modernity) is a post-traditional order where 'the self, like the broader institutional contexts in which it exists, has to be reflexively made' (1991: 3). Giddens claims that in late modernity the globalising tendencies of modern institutions are accompanied by a transformation of day-to-day social life which, in turn, has profound implications for personal activities. In particular, the dynamism characteristic of modern institutional life undercuts traditional habits and customs; there is a 'disembedding of social institutions' which interlaces in a direct way with individual life and therefore self (Giddens 1991: 1).

For Giddens, the diminution of traditional social formations leads to a reduction in indigenous forms of social control and an increasing emphasis on self discovery through a multiplicity of lifestyle choices. Giddens argues that the conditions of late modernity have important implications for psychic processes as well as the body. 'The reflexivity of the self extends to the body, where the body is part of an action system rather than merely a passive object' (Giddens 1991: 77). For him the body is 'reflexively mobilised', available to be 'worked upon' by the influences of high modernity (Giddens 1991: 218). This self-reflexive process generates lifestyle planning and 'bodily regimes' which are, he argues, 'generic to the circumstances of day-to-day life' (Giddens 1991: 105).

The historical framework of this argument about the body and self as a project could be criticised: religion, for example, has long been implicated in such processes (Turner 1996: 21). Similarly, the elusiveness of a gendered self-identity and the historical significance of bodily control in constructing a sense of masculinity over the past two centuries in North American culture are well documented (Kimmel 1994). Other criticisms include Giddens' analytic focus on future oriented minds and a failure to recognise that identity may be tied to an embodied *habitus* (Shilling and Mellor 1996). Indeed, the body as a practical accomplishment, constituted through ongoing choices, may be made unreflexively through habit. Nevertheless, despite certain limitations, Giddens (1991) usefully draws attention to the plasticity of the mobile, embodied and reflexive self in a global context of innovative but potentially risky health technologies.

Late modernity, according to Giddens (1991) and also Beck (1992), is essentially a risk-oriented world where selves, and bodies, have to be reflexively constructed and mobilised amidst continuous warnings about danger. Historically speaking life has always been 'risky' but contemporary risks have profoundly altered as a consequence of human interventions (Williams and Bendelow 1998: 104–5). Warnings about manufactured, imperceptible and globalised danger abound, but within late modernity there are no determinant 'authorities' (at least, not in the traditional sense) with which to evaluate competing knowledge claims (Giddens 1991: 194). The fracturing of any consensus about what represents 'expert' opinion, as noted by Green (1997a: 457), prompts late modern individuals to assume increasing responsibility in assessing their own risk environment. Considerations of risk may be filtered through contact with expert knowledge

(Giddens 1991: 5) but a myriad of other sources, including ubiquitous 'guides to living' (i.e. books and manuals), provide information instrumental in the reflexive construction of the self and the body (Nettleton and Watson 1998: 6).

Important work on the sociology of the body is identifiable but much of this literature is theoretically driven and is empirically lacking. After reviewing Giddens (1991), specifically the alleged pliability of bodies, and people's active attempts to alter, improve and refine them, Nettleton and Watson (1998: 7) highlight the need for empirical investigation using a phenomenological approach. That is, an empirically grounded approach concerned with human 'embodiment' (Nettleton and Watson 1998: 9): a concept which 'more adequately captures the notions of making and doing the work of bodies – of becoming bodies in social space' (Turner 1996: xiii). Others bemoan the dearth of empirical evidence with which to test corporeal claims and analytical insights. Williams and Bendelow (1998: 104) write: 'Discourses on risk, consumption and the "reflexive" body [...] continue to be pitched, for the most part, at the level of broad claims and sweeping generalisations with little concern for empirical detail ...'

From a theoretical stance it could be argued that bodybuilding represents a 'risky' lifestyle choice for sustaining a coherent narrative of self-identity, an *opportunity* for transformation (*cf.* Fox 1998: 683–4) and a function of the openness of the future (and the body) to colonisation (Giddens 1991, Scott *et al.* 1998). Moreover, bodybuilders, who are steroid users, are engaging in chemical, not just social, constructions; hence, it could be posited that the beneficial possibilities of science and technology are double edged, creating new parameters of risk (Giddens 1991: 27–8). Here the project-like activity of bodybuilding represents a substantive topic suitable for detailed empirical investigation. A grounded study of bodybuilding offers the potential to investigate and link formal sociological concerns with embodiment, identity, gender and risk. Relevant questions include: to what extent do new social parameters of risk and body modification traverse the sex/gender system? Sociologists of health and medicine, for example, suggest traditional conceptions of gender *may* be insignificant in constructing perfect bodies through risky medical technologies (Annandale 1998: 80).

Giddens (1991) work on reflexive bodies should not be viewed in isolation. Academic literature on the body and self-identity is now voluminous, incorporating a host of perspectives derived from various disciplines (Shilling 1993). A study of bodybuilding, drugs and risk must recognise and reference these largely theoretical contributions. For example, the biomedical model of the 'naturalistic' body – although reductionistic and overly deterministic – undoubtedly shapes Western understandings of physicality and is therefore sociologically relevant (Frank 1990). Many bodybuilders' ability to experience and theorise about the material body – including their subcultural knowledge of genetics, drug (side) effects and possible behavioural changes attendant to steroid abuse – is inextricably medicalised. There is also important anthropological work on techniques of the body (Mauss 1973), ethnophysiological understandings (Manning and Fabrega 1973), indigenous body modification practices (Brain 1979), diet and the cultural construction of identity (Borre 1991). This empirical literature, which partly compensates for sociology's long-standing neglect of bodily matters, facilitates comparative analysis of bodybuilders' self-presentation, embodied perceptions, knowledge and practices. Similarly, feminist scholars usefully underscore the significance of gender and power on women's interactions with new body technologies (Balsamo 1996). Space constraints prohibit a review of this literature. However, insights from these materials, along with other important work (e.g. Bourdieu *et al.* 1991, Crossley 1995, Elias 1978, Foucault 1986, Goffman 1968, Merleau-Ponty 1962, Turner 1992), are included.

Bodybuilding subculture

While bodybuilding is a highly gendered (male dominated) activity, aspects of the enterprise, similar to fitness more generally, may be considered postmodern by blurring the male-female dichotomy (Fussell 1994, Glassner 1990). However, bodybuilding may at one level challenge a straightforward gender dichotomy but it also (somewhat paradoxically) reproduces the heterobinarism of the sex/gender system (Lowe 1998). Powerful (sub)cultural discourses construct 'natural' hetero-sexual gender differences within bodybuilding and sociological literature in this area typically adopts a dichotomous analysis. Correspondingly, this section of the literature review is structured according to a heterobinary logic.

Critical feminist work on male bodybuilding is first considered. In particular, critical attention is directed at Klein (1993), who, at the time of this research, had published the only ethnographic monograph on this subject. Literature on female bodybuilding and drug use is then noted.

Critical feminist studies of male bodybuilding

Recent work in men's studies claim that Western culture is experiencing a crisis-in-masculinity, rendering many men unsure about their masculine identities. With taken-for-granted notions of culturally dominant (hegemonic) masculinity being challenged in many social spheres (e.g. the workplace and family), sport is believed to represent one strategy for retaining, continuing and reproducing hegemonic masculinity (White and Gillett 1994: 20). It is argued that bodybuilding in particular provides men (and some women suffering personal insecurities) with an atavistic means of redressing their feelings of powerlessness through the pursuit of a culturally valorised mesomorphic image signifying hegemonic masculinity. Here bodybuilding, drugs and risk are attributed to the dual interplay of antecedent psychological and sociocultural forces perceived to be beyond individual control (Gillett and White 1992, Klein 1995).

If 'the muscular body' is located within mainstream normative limits (i.e. if it approximates the athletically fit-looking body valorised in consumer culture), then muscularity clearly denotes (among other things) power and self-control. These qualities undoubtedly feed into dominant conceptions of masculinity within patriarchal society (Klein 1993: 242), and have been linked to a variety of risk behaviours in the health field (Sabo and Gordon 1995). Critical feminists maintain that because bodybuilding superficially presents an image of power conforming to hegemonic masculinity, the subculture ineffectively compensates for members' feelings of insecurity and low self-esteem. The basis for asserting bodybuilding is 'hyper-masculine' and an atavistic compensatory mechanism for personal and gender inadequacy is elaborated below before offering some possible criticisms.

Historical determinations inscribe on the body masculinity and femininity. This is due to the sexual division of labour where muscularity is relegated to the functioning of the body (physical labour) thus underwriting morphological differences between men and women (Klein 1993: 5). Klein adds that historically men defined themselves through participation in traditional occupations requiring physical strength. A corollary being that within our society 'muscles (and the building of them) are a standard that men feel compelled to strive for, rationalize, repudiate, or otherwise dismiss. Women simply do not have to deal with muscles in so compulsory a manner' (Klein 1993: 6). However, the *presumed* role of bodybuilding in achieving a progressive sense of masculinity is flawed according to critical feminists. Klein (1993) notes that industrialisation has rendered obsolete physically strenuous and demanding occupations which traditionally served as a source of masculine identity. Hence, because form is separated from function (musculature is less important for the economically functioning body) under such conditions 'muscles, for those who readily define themselves by them, become emblematic of a masculinity in crisis' (1993: 6).

Social scientific work demonstrates unequivocally that masculinity is socially constructed (Connell 1995) and that changes in economic production have rendered the active, sporting body (created, for example, through vigorous workouts with barbells and prescribed tonics) historically central in such processes (Kimmel

1994: 26). Contemporary bodybuilding, like its nineteenth-century fledgling 'Physical Culture', enables male participants to accrue gender imbued muscle and embody ideals linked to masculinity such as competence and force (Jefferson 1998). Similarly, the emphasis in bodybuilding on autonomy, rationality, control and discipline has strong masculine connotations in Western culture. Undoubtedly, the social construction of masculinity may *contribute* to the current appeal and sustainability of bodybuilding, given a social structural shift in gender relations and the erosion of traditional sources of masculine identity. However, while social structure is significant, especially when studying the social dynamics of risk (Hart and Flowers 1996), as commented by Whitehead when reviewing recent work on hegemonic masculinity: 'macro-structuralist interpretations can only reveal so much' (1999: 61). Correspondingly, it is legitimate to ask whether the ongoing variable and potentially 'risky' project of bodybuilding can be adequately theorised in terms of social structural changes and the construction of hegemonic masculinity?

One possible criticism is that the sexual division of labour, even in parts of Britain experiencing a shrinking manufacturing base (e.g. South Wales), may remain a source of gender identity for some bodybuilders. As Klein (1993) recognises, most bodybuilders have to work to support their training, and are employed in a *range* of occupations. These include types of work where strength is advantageous (though being a bodybuilder is not requisite for such work) and where, especially in relation to the validation of masculine identity, the body is 'risked in performance' (Jefferson 1998). For example, women continue to be highly marginalised in jobs such as fire-fighting and night club security work. This suggests there may be other (more fundamental?) reasons for bodybuilding, aside from possible insecurities associated with a man's position in the division of labour. Furthermore, the importance of finance for successful bodybuilding (see Chapter 3) counters the commonsense assumption that muscle-building is a pursuit favoured by unemployed men in search of a secure masculine identity. Regular consumption of bodybuilding technologies is dependent upon material security and advantage, factors associated with self-control and mastery. These points certainly do not invalidate the masculinity-in-crisis thesis, but they do lead one to question its generality when accounting for individual involvement in bodybuilding.

Other criticisms may be made, relating specifically to the critical feminist claim that bodybuilders endeavour to embody a mesomorphic image signifying hegemonic masculinity. Do 1990s bodybuilders really embody a culturally valorised body-image, rendering bodybuilding a late modern reassertion of hegemonic masculinity? It is clear to the bodybuilding cognoscenti that the types of muscular body which today's muscle enthusiasts create physically differ from

9

the traditional masculinist model of physicality. Former bodybuilder Sam Fussell writes: 'Those who actually work with their bodies don't look remotely like body-builders, whether it be the village smithy or farmers' (1994: 44). Moreover, if modern day competition standard bodybuilding physiques are considered stigmatising by non-initiates (including weight trainers on the margins of bodybuilding subculture), then social process in the affiliative context of bodybuilding is important when accounting for individual commitment to the cult of muscularity. Rather than being antecedent, motives and dispositions for *transmogrifying* the body emerge during the course of experience within a subcultural context (*cf.* Becker 1963).

The previous critical point is worth elaborating. Existing theoretical work pays scant attention to the heterogeneity of bodybuilding. 'The muscular body', fashioned through bodywork, is mainly understood as a singular as opposed to a plural concept. However, in differentiating types of muscular body which are homogenous to non-participants, neophytes learn to decipher the 'artistic merits' of types of bodybuilding physique which are stigmatised (not valorised) outside of bodybuilding subculture. Bodybuilders' 'pictorial competence', learnt through habit and exercise (Bourdieu *et al.* 1991: 109) in the bodybuilding habitus, effec-tively becomes a basis of choice and a motivating structure (see Crossley 1995, Shilling 1993). This does not mean that the sex/gender system is irrelevant in shaping and constraining choice, and gender anxieties may still figure in the genesis and continuation of bodywork for a proportion of bodybuilders. However, anteced-ent insecurities are neither a necessary nor sufficient condition for bodybuilding.

To be sure, critical feminist studies are not irrelevant. For example, White and Gillett (1994: 28–30) usefully describe how male bodybuilders disavow the passivity of being looked at, or, more specifically, how they avoid the risk of feminisation. Male bodybuilders, as noted in this literature, adopt strategies that maintain the idea of masculinity-as-activity, including aggressive poses when displaying their bodies for the camera. Also, Klein (1993) provides important insights into, among other things, bodybuilders' argot and symbolic style, cultural relations with the larger society and possible psychosocial factors promoting a predilection to bodybuilding. Nevertheless, while sociologically valuable, these constructivist accounts do not offer detailed ethnographic analyses which address the sustainability and variability of (chemical) bodybuilding. The blind spots and limitations of critical feminist studies of bodybuilding may be attributed to a priori political commitments, a tendency to relegate human agency to outside forces, and, specifically in respect of Klein's (1993) ethnography, his methodology.

In emphasising the importance of methodological sensitivity, qualitative researchers studying male bodies and health, employ 'grounded theory [which produces] definitions of reality that are inherently valid, verifiable and applicable' (Watson 2000: 8). Various methodological criticisms may be levelled against Klein (1993), using the grounded theory approach (Glaser and Strauss 1967). First, there is the implicit assurance that there were plenty of data which verify his theoretical claims (Klein 1993: 282). However, in mainly presenting well-tested theory fragments concerning the significance of antecedent insecurities in bodybuilding, Klein (1993) can only partially account for what is happening in the researched situation (Glaser and Strauss 1967: 27). Second, Klein (1993) does not include a sufficient range of cases in his analysis. In confining his study to elite bodybuilders, he limits the possibility of comparison between and among groups within the same empirical field. Third, one way of ensuring the credibility of qualitative research is to use a codified procedure for analysing data (Glaser and Strauss 1967: 229). This allows readers to understand how the analyst obtained their theory from the data. Because Klein (1993) apparently eschews a coded method of analysis (he makes no reference to using a coded procedure for handling his voluminous data) one cannot help feeling that his theoretical interpretations can be anything but impressionistic (see Glaser and Strauss 1967: 229).

Other criticisms may be levelled, and alternative theories invoked to account for the widespread appeal of leisure pursuits in general and bodybuilding in particular. For instance, writings on the sociology of the body (which, similar to critical feminism, largely remain at the level of abstracted affinities) cite the growth of visually oriented consumer culture in 'post-industrial' society and the contemporary emphasis on keeping fit, the body beautiful and the postponement of ageing by sport (Turner 1991a). Similarly, literature on the *representational* significance of the exercised and dieted fe/male body within postmodernity (Glassner 1990) offer equally satisfactory ways of theorising bodybuilding and drug-taking independent of a masculinity-in-crisis. For example, if positive health is conceived in representational rather than instrumental terms, and the image of health has become more real than the 'real' thing it references, then 'anomalous' activities such as drug 'abuse' are understandable. This literature cannot be reviewed here, but the possibility of alternative (though not entirely incompatible) readings of bodybuilding and drug-taking should be recognised.

Drug use and femininity

Difficulties in getting athletes to be open about their drug use means that researchers have obtained 'only a glimpse of a huge underground subculture' (Yesalis 1992: 16). Correspondingly, sociologists studying bodybuilding have mainly addressed gender issues rather than drug use specifically. However, drug use is of central significance. As well as health considerations, drug-taking in bodybuilding subculture is mediated by notions concerning the degree to which muscularity is an acceptable aspect of feminine/masculine appearance. The limited research on drug-taking among bodybuilders focuses primarily on men. Klein's (1995) paper on steroid use among male bodybuilders is indicative of a more general neglect of drug use among female bodybuilders. It is to be recognised that research in this area is difficult not least because women drug-using bodybuilders comprise a small minority of gym members. And, while this may be partly compensated by a high prevalence of steroid use, female athletes may be hesitant to disclose their use to researchers because steroids often produce 'embarrassing' secondary male sexual characteristics (Strauss and Yesalis 1993: 153–4). Women taking steroids 'risk' irreversible virilising effects including excessive facial and body hair and deepening of the voice. It is conceivable that some women may welcome these (side?) effects for purposes of transgressing traditional sex/gender constructs. However, the dominant meanings of these social risks render steroid use especially problematic for many female bodybuilders whose bodies and identities are forged in a (sub)culture that seeks to naturalise gender differences.

To be sure, social scientists have not totally ignored the use of drugs among female bodybuilders and recent ethnographic work provides some useful data. Lowe (1998), in particular, discusses the social aspects of steroid use in female bodybuilding, focusing upon the relationship between femininity, muscularity and signs of steroid use. While there are a variety of views on this within bodybuilding, the perceived 'inappropriateness' of steroid use is largely explicable in terms of the masculinist connotations of 'excessive' muscularity (Lowe 1998: 75). These hegemonic ideologies are implicated in processes and strategies rendering female bodybuilders less threatening to the 'natural' gender order. Possible constraints on steroid use among women, such as negative (sub)cultural evaluations, are significant. Other recuperative strategies include the fashioning of moderately muscular (culturally acceptable/desirable Ms Figure-Fitness) types of body (Schulze 1990, St Martin and Gavey 1996). These lesser muscular bodies, displayed at Fitness/Figure competitions, are favoured by many people who are critical of steroid use among women (Lowe 1998). Here, as in other domains, 'appropriate' feminine bodies and identities are produced and shaped by heterosexual imperatives (Jackson 1996).

The relationship between muscularity, femininity and steroids is discussed in recent sociological literature. However, women bodybuilders' potential and actual use of different physique-enhancing drugs, the specificities and ethnopharmacological rationale for taking and avoiding various substances (including types of steroid) is relatively unexplored territory. Strauss and Yesalis' (1993) paper examining the additional effects of steroids on women, for example, does not describe bodybuilders' gendered drug repertoires, women's differential risk management strategies and the construction of competent social identities. Gendered knowledge and drug use patterns are verbalised by (non-)steroid-using male and female bodybuilders and are crystallised in subcultural pharmacopoeia. These accounts of 'gender appropriate' risk-taking behaviour, similar to accounts offered by Green's respondents (1997b: 188), suggest that a gendered identity may be achieved through talk about risk (if not actual risk-taking).

In discussing bodybuilding, drugs and risk more generally, literature published by researchers from a range of disciplines and practices is relevant. Although this literature largely focuses upon steroid use, bodybuilders' sophisticated use of other drugs is recognised. In remaining eclectic it is therefore possible to identify some academic work reporting bodybuilders' complex drug-taking practices. For example, Evans (1997) and Pates and Barry (1996), survey the drug-taking habits of steroid users in South Wales, revealing that combinations of drugs were common. Research conducted among professional calibre bodybuilders in the USA provides similar findings (Augé and Augé 1999). Other research conducted among steroid users in the North West of England (Lenehan et al. 1996) also notes types of drug combined with steroids and other relevant background information. For instance, they identify the most commonly used steroids, note most steroid users inject, underscore the importance of needle exchange facilities and document self-reported physical and psychological side effects. Admittedly, rich qualitative data are not reported and analysed in these studies. Nevertheless, this literature underscores the need for more detailed research specifically on bodybuilders' ethnopharmacological knowledge, risk management strategies and negotiation of self-identity.

Papers written by social workers, psychologists, psychiatrists and other medical researchers are identifiable (e.g. Burgess 1993, McKillop 1987, Pope and Katz 1990). This literature – which identifies, or rather constructs, bodybuilders, recreational gym members, adolescent males and others as 'at risk' – is largely concerned with the 'improper' use of medicines, and physical and behavioural drug side effects. Similarly, the fairly comprehensive collection of writings edited by Yesalis (1993) is explicitly correctionalist and only offers a scant understanding of bodybuilders' drug-taking methods and rationale as understood by bodybuilders themselves (cf. Gilbert 1993: xxv).

Sociological literature on drug use in bodybuilding, as noted in relation to female bodybuilders, is underdeveloped. Goldstein (1990) provides a valuable ethnographic overview of steroid use among US gym members, but such work is largely introductory in scope. This dearth is surprising given the centrality of drugs in bodybuilding (Klein 1986: 122–4). Although Klein (1986) acknowledges the significance of steroid-taking, and his later monograph mentions the use of Human Growth Hormone and Thyroid medication (1993: 147–52), the intricacies of bodybuilding ethnopharmacology are not central to such work. Others such as Gillett and White (1992: 366) simply mention steroid use in bodybuilding as an aside, writing that 'the health risks of using anabolic steroids can be serious [making] the strategy of bodybuilding an ultimately fatal one'. More recent work on steroid use (Klein 1995) takes a similar line, reiterating dominant medical understandings, viz. that these drugs are necessarily 'hazardous' to mind, body and public safety. Such work, in perceiving risk through an egalitarian filter that assigns minimal significance to benefits (Adams 1995), does not detail body-builders' complex understandings which sustain and legitimate drug use over time. Instead, steroid use and the 'inherent' dangers of the activity are taken to bolster the claim that bodybuilding is a subculture characterised by inadequacy.

This book contributes to the literature by detailing bodybuilders' sophisticated ethnopharmacological knowledge of, and experimentation with, various physique-enhancing drugs. Treating drug-taking as rational and responsive to social context (see Bloor 1995: 91), it documents how subcultural affiliation influences bodybuilders' social construction of hazards, risk perceptions and risk-management strategies. Correspondingly, this study recognises that behaviours labelled as risk-inducing – while frequently remaining unconsidered and taken-for-granted among individuals routinely engaging in such activities (Schutz 1970) – may also be sustained by 'lay' actors who consider themselves competent and who challenge experts' definitions of hazards and risks. From one perspective the inherently risky use of drugs among bodybuilders represents a 'knee-jerk' response to a masculinity-in-crisis (Klein 1993, 1995). Alternatively, chemical bodybuilding is 'symptomatic' of a more general questioning of authority, expertise and professionalism in late modernity (*cf.* Gabe *et al.* 1994).

Steroids and violence

A study of bodybuilding, drugs and risk cannot ignore the commonly perceived link between steroids and violence. For bodybuilders the central characteristic of steroids is their capacity to enhance physique and performance. However, increased aggression, or, more specifically, uncontrollable outbursts of anger known as 'Roid-Rage, has been described by scientific observers as the central defining effect of steroids (Riem and Hursey 1995: 249). Here concerns about risks to steroid users' health are substituted by concerns for public safety (Lubell 1989) and/or the safety of female partners of male steroid users (Choi and Pope 1994).

Medical and behavioural science literature, describing possible psychiatric and behavioural steroid effects, is reviewed below. The primary intention here is to document prevalent *ideas* on this topic rather than discuss the methodological limitations of specific studies. Reference is first made to writings lending scientific support to the 'Roid-Rage phenomenon (e.g. Pope and Katz 1990). Scientific literature also encompasses work where 'researchers have questioned both the prevalence of negative effects (e.g. Bahrke, Yesalis, & Wright, 1990; Perry, Yates, & Anderson, 1990) and their hypothesized pharmacological basis, suggesting that responses to AAS [steroid] administration may be partially mediated by the self-fulfilment of expectations about AASs' effects (Bjorkqvist, Nygren, Bjorklund, & Bjorkqvist, 1994; Cicero & O'Connor, 1990), by users' perceptions of their changing physique and performance (Brower, Blow, Young, and Hill, 1991; Yesalis *et al.*, 1990), or by personality traits (Moss, Panzak and Tarter, 1992; Yates, Perry, & Anderson, 1990)' (Riem and Hursey 1995: 235–6). Some of these other studies, which question the 'malevolence assumption' (Hamilton and Collins 1981) under-pinning much steroid research, are also reviewed. Finally, no systematic effort is made to distinguish aggression from violence. This is because the steroids-violence literature generally conflates mood and behaviour (Goldstein and Lee 1994: 3).

According to one contributor to the 'Roid-Rage perspective: 'steroids may result in significant adverse psychiatric effects and behavioural changes [and] some of these effects may result in violent criminal behaviour' (Uzych 1992: 23). Others posit a more deterministic relationship (e.g. Brower *et al.* 1994, Choi and Pope 1994), positing either activational versions of the 'Roid-Rage hypothesis (i.e. immediate/slightly delayed drug effects) or organisational versions (*cf.* Kashkin 1992, Riem and Hursey 1995). The latter, less common variant of the theory, maintains that steroids cause long-lasting changes in brain morphology, dysfunctional reasoning and negative behaviours which are independent of subsequent hormone activity (Riem and Hursey 1995: 240). In implicitly referring to the more popular activational version of the 'Roid-Rage hypothesis, Williamson writes: 'despite numerous reports of violent behaviour among anabolic steroid users there is little scientific evidence that the use of anabolic steroids actually causes aggression' (1994: 20). Nevertheless, the dominant idea expressed by science is that there is a definite correlation between current/past steroid-taking and aggressive violence. The link is not always cast as direct and causal but the general consensus is that there is an association.

Riem and Hursey examine the relevant scientific literature on this topic. In a context where 'concern has been raised that persons using anabolic-androgenic steroids may experience negative psychological states', these authors refer to activational accounts in order to 'evaluate theory based hypotheses regarding AAS-mood and behaviour associations' (1995: 235). Importantly, they state that although the issue is of current scientific interest, research on the topic is scant:

> Debate among experts as to how AASs affect psychological functioning and the significance of their effects for psychosocial adjustment reflects not only increased scientific interest in the non-medical use of AAS but also limitations of the research base.
>
> (Riem and Hursey 1995: 236)

Although research on the non-medical use of steroids is limited, relevant here is the observation that 'most research assessing the affective and behavioural changes athletes encounter has taken the "'roid-rage" perspective, looking for negative outcomes accompanying AAS' (Riem and Hursey 1995: 236). Riem and Hursey add: 'this negative pharmacological conceptualisation has biased the current literature by implicitly excluding many mediators and outcomes from consideration' (1995: 236). Although biased, this literature informs popular and media discourse on steroid effects. Furthermore, current research contributes to the set of expectations surrounding possible behavioural side effects. Thus, what do specific studies say about steroids and aggressive violence?

Choi *et al.* (1989) claim that alterations in mood and behaviour occur among persons while consuming steroids, and accompanying negative psychological/ behavioural changes are the direct result of pharmacological processes involving neurochemical systems. Adopting a negative pharmacological conceptualisation, Choi *et al.* (1989) briefly review what they consider the adverse behavioural effects of steroids in athletes. Reference is made to clinical studies, case histories and scientific experimental data to examine the supposed steroid activational effects on behaviour. For these authors, steroid-behaviour links are directly caused by altering the levels of sex hormones (1989: 183):

> High dose anabolic steroids are often found to lead to increased aggression and hostility. This is particularly noticeable following multiple high drug use or 'stacking'. Psychotic symptoms also occur and researchers have noted a connection between stacking and violent assault, attempted murder or actual murder. Upon drug withdrawal these behavioural changes generally reverse but may be accompanied by feelings of depression.

Choi *et al.* (1989) acknowledge that their findings are far from conclusive. Nevertheless they add: 'though the primary interest of anabolic steroid research to date has focused on the medical and physiological effects, the present review illustrates that behaviour change can be very pronounced and in some cases alarming' (1989: 186).

In 'Homicide and Near-Homicide by Anabolic Steroid Users', Pope and Katz (1990) present a similar account. For these authors steroids activate the central nervous system causing increased irritability and aggressiveness (1990: 28). They write that results published from their previous study, supporting this conceptualisation, were widely quoted in the popular press. This, in turn, elicited inquiries from lawyers and attorneys, each describing an individual who had apparently committed a violent crime while taking steroids. After following up three of these cases, Pope and Katz (1990) present case reports supporting their hypothesis that steroids exert activational effects causing aggressive violence. Concerning their view that steroids represent the principle aetiology for the psychiatric symptoms and criminal behaviour described, they write: 'These three cases strongly suggest that anabolic steroids may cause some law-abiding and psychiatrically asymptomatic individuals to develop manic and psychotic symptoms, culminating occasionally in violent crimes' (1990: 30).

Undoubtedly, some bodybuilders may find the 'steroid defence' (Moss 1988) useful as an excuse for untoward conduct. However, bodybuilders contacted during this research often resisted these deterministic propositions. In legitimating their drug activities, bodybuilders rejected steroids as an exculpatory discourse by 'denying injury' to others (Weinstein 1980). This vocabulary of motive, concordant with the rationalised and consciously restrained 'civilised body' (Elias 1978), is understandable. The uncritical acceptance of 'Roid-Rage could have negative ideological implications for members of this drug subculture. Irrespective of personal use, bodybuilders would have to concede that their subculturally normalised drug-taking practices were 'socially problematic'. While accepting testosterone derivatives may enhance or exaggerate aggressive feelings, bodybuilders resisted scientific 'truths' by modifying various versions of the 'Roid-Rage hypothesis. They distinguished aggression from violence, and argued other factors are as equally significant as the drugs themselves, including: users' expectations about steroid effects, perceptions which users (especially new users and newcomers to bodybuilding) have of their changing physique and performance, alongside the personality traits of some users (*cf.* Riem and Hursey 1995: 235–6). Furthermore, many bodybuilders resisted the straightforward association between steroids and aggression/violence given the heterogeneity of steroids, variations in dosages, drug combinations and contextual factors mediating between mood change and aggressive violence. Similar ideas have been expressed by researchers who question both the prevalence of negative effects and their hypothesised pharmacological basis.

Bjorkqvist *et al.* (1994) suggest that responses to steroid administration may be partially mediated by the self-fulfilment of expectations about steroid effects. For these authors, there is a clear placebo effect. In their double blind experiment, subjects who were given a placebo, somewhat surprisingly, became more irritable, frustrated and angry than those who were given testosterone and a control group receiving no treatment. In referring to the literature, they add: 'Two recent studies investigating the relationship between anabolic-androgenic steroid use and mood changes (Anderson *et al.* 1992, Bahrke *et al.* 1992) yielded the same result as the present experiment: Steroid intake did not increase aggressiveness in human males' (Bjorkqvist *et al.* 1994: 24; also, see Bhasin *et al.* 1996, who administer a significantly higher dosage and report similar findings). They write: 'to claim [...] aggression is caused by steroids, as in the news media, is misleading and dangerous for several reasons' (Bjorkqvist *et al.* 1994: 25). Three reasons are given for rejecting the popular claim that steroids cause aggression. Namely, there is still no scientific evidence for such a relationship; even if there was a correlation this would not prove a cause-effect relationship; and finally, such a claim is dangerous because:

> Dissemination of the myth of the steroid-aggressiveness connection may lead to anticipation (a placebo effect) of aggressiveness among steroid abusers and, in turn, to actual acts of violence. It may, in fact, work as an excuse for aggression.
>
> (Bjorkqvist *et al.* 1994: 25)

Similar to alcohol, steroids may represent a socially sanctioned opportunity to take 'Time-Out', thus excusing unacceptable behaviour (Macandrew and Edgerton 1970). This, of course, has more to do with common sociocultural ideas – complicit with a hierarchical gender order which 'naturalises' male domination – than the psychopharmacological properties of the drugs themselves (Bjorkqvist *et al.* 1994: 25). Possible behaviour changes accompanying steroid use may be seen to be unrelated to the steroids per se but would be an expectancy effect (Riem and Hursey 1995: 239).

In noting factors which mediate individual responses to steroids, Riem and Hursey (1995: 235–6) mention users' self-perceptions and beliefs concerning their changing physiques. Although Brower *et al.* (1991) and Yesalis *et al.* (1990) are cited as researchers providing some supportive evidence, they write: 'in sum, almost no data on self-perceptions exist' (Riem and Hursey 1995: 251). This gap in the research persists 'even though anecdotal reports suggest almost all AAS users experience physique and performance changes' (Riem and Hursey 1995: 251). Concerning the supposed behavioural effects of steroids, in addition to rationalisations for continued use, bodybuilders' self-perceptions are relevant. Indeed, if 'increased libido or energy induced by AAS are pleasurable, users' [self-esteem] should increase as well. If, however, higher sex steroid activity is unpleasant, then athletes should have lower self-images while using AAS' (Riem and Hursey 1995: 250). Implications for resultant behaviour are clear. For instance, if a bodybuilder using steroids has improved self-esteem, body-image and perceived competencies in specific social or physical domains (Riem and Hursey 1995: 250) then they may become more assertive in social interaction, or behave in a way which may be interpreted as aggressive (similarly, see Goldstein and Lee 1994: 6). As Riem and Hursey (1995) point out, few studies provide data relevant to such questions. Reference to their work therefore usefully highlights existing limitations in the research base. This study, in investigating (steroid-using) bodybuilders' understandings, prioritises self-related perceptions and knowledge thus helping to redress this gap in the literature.

The research

Most of the data were generated and prepared for formal analysis between 1994 and 1996, during an 'Economic and Social Research Council' funded project. Using ethnography, depth interviews, and materials from secondary sources (e.g. international bodybuilding magazines, steroid handbooks, published insider accounts), the research sought specifically to investigate supposed bodybuilding-steroids-violence associations. However, bodybuilding, drugs and risk more generally were subjected to detailed empirical investigation, thereby providing rich qualitative data for this study.

Researching international materials (and interviewing bodybuilders from outside of Wales) leads me to propose that this study's findings extend beyond South Wales, and that bodybuilders' 'risky' identities and practices involve the articulation of global cultural discourses which (in the affluent developed world) cut across bounded societies and states (Giddens 1991). Nevertheless, given critical feminist arguments on bodybuilding, the study's geographic location is noteworthy. According to Harris (1987), mining and steel production have been powerful determinants of masculinity and gender relations in South Wales. In the past two decades this part of Britain has experienced a shrinking manufacturing base, a diminution of traditional male working patterns of employment and a marginal, though socially significant, increase in the employment opportunities for women (Cooke 1987). One aspect of this research, therefore, was to empirically examine whether the 'fatal' strategy of bodybuilding (Gillett and White 1992) could be adequately theorised in terms of antecedent insecurities caused by a 'masculinity-in-crisis' and a wish to embody the physical trappings of hegemonic masculinity (Klein 1993).

While undertaking pilot work, fifteen bodybuilding gyms, twelve leisure centres, three needle exchanges and a Well Steroid User Clinic were surveyed in twelve towns located across South Wales. Participant observation was also undertaken at physique competitions and various other settings e.g. night clubs, respondents' homes, 'gyms' in back street garages. Commercial bodybuilding gyms were eventually selected as the main ethnographic site, and the main ethnographic study was conducted on a time-sampling basis at four gyms over a sixteen month period. These gyms (Olympia, Al's Gym, Pumping Iron and The Temple) were identified as 'hard core' by bodybuilders, meaning they had the requisite equipment and atmosphere associated with the serious business of creating 'the perfect body'.

As noted, researchers have cited difficulties in investigating drug use among bodybuilders (Pates and Barry 1996). As an ethnography, access difficulties were minimised by regularly participating in gym culture over an extended period and obtaining the assistance of a 'locator' (Soccer) who made proper introductions (similarly, see Stewart-Clevidence and Goldstein 1996: 36). Given the sensitive nature of the research, contacts were assured of anonymity. They were told names and certain details specific to particular gyms and individuals would be changed or omitted in subsequent reports to avoid possible identification.

Anthropologists undertaking ethnopharmacological studies among non-Western peoples highlight the possibility of obtaining indigenous understandings, even when members are considered secretive (Etkin 1993). Of course, as a 'reflexive' ethnographer I recognise the significance of researcher characteristics, especially when studying so-called 'deviant' groups (Hammersley and Atkinson 1995). For example, social access, or rather, my ability to 'get on' and generate data in this male dominated subculture, was facilitated by my male gender, my adoption of a physically demanding but potentially stigmatising 'active membership role' (Adler and Adler 1987), and accompanying bodily changes. My active and ongoing participation in gym culture – sustained by a personal interest in sport, exercise and active lifestyles – may signal a reverse of the 'halo effect' enjoyed by researchers studying high status groups. However, as Goffman

(1989: 125) argues, ethnography entails submitting one's personality, social situation and body (within certain limits) to the set of contingencies that play upon individuals comprising the studied collectivity. (See Monaghan, 1999a, for a more detailed account of the study methodology.)

As well as ethnographic fieldwork, qualitative data were generated using a detailed interview schedule. Given the work-oriented nature of bodybuilding gyms this was a particularly valuable research tool. As well as establishing my identity as an academic researcher, it represented a useful opportunity to take 'time out' from bodybuilders' more immediate practical concerns. Often, topics addressed during lengthy audio-recorded face-to-face interviews (some of which were held over several days, lasting in excess of six hours) related to matters that were not casually topical, but sociologically relevant (similarly, see Holstein and Gubrium 1997: 126). These phenomenologically open interviews provided detailed qualitative data on various issues including: orientations to lifting weights; diverse sources of information; bodybuilders' ethno-pharmacological, nutritional and physiological knowledge; risk perceptions and management strategies.

These interview data, which facilitate comparative analysis and the enrichment of emergent theories (Glaser and Strauss 1967: 68–9), are quoted in this study verbatim. They occupy a complementary role to fieldwork materials gathered during participant observation (Silverman 1993). It should be noted that data source and non-personal identifiers (pseudonyms and/or interview numbers), which establish context of data production and which differentiate speakers while preserving anonymity, are attached to excerpts in ensuing empirical chapters. If quotes have been edited to avoid repetition or altered in order fully to express their sense, then ellipses [...] are used.

Sixty-seven in-depth interviews were conducted using the schedule between 1994 and 1995. In attempting to obtain a theoretically representative sample – which is necessary in the generation of theory and a wider understanding of social processes (Glaser and Strauss 1967) – a range of bodybuilders and weight trainers were interviewed. Most respondents were recruited through ethnographic contacts, though others were contacted including a group of men (N=15) who exercised with weights in a prison. (Not all of my informal ethnographic contacts were interviewed with the schedule. Some, for example, who were willing to talk to me in gyms could not afford the time to be 'formally' interviewed.) Posters were also placed in three needle exchange facilities, and an advertisement was featured in a British bodybuilding magazine. These mediated contact strategies were not very successful, resulting in only three additional interviews.

In noting some general characteristics of the interview sample, forty reported using or ever using steroids (60 per cent) and twenty-seven claimed to have never used. Bodybuilders comprised a significant proportion of the sample (N=40 or 60 per cent). Three quarters of all bodybuilders interviewed (N=30) said they used or had used steroids. Regarding the competition status of bodybuilders, 60 per cent (N=24) had entered a physique show. These competitions ranged from the local level to world championship standard. The interviews primarily involved male respondents, though six women were recruited (9 per cent of the sample). One of these women, who was married to a male steroid injector, took steroids and was of International competitive standard in the Ms Physique category (women aiming for maximum muscle mass and definition). Another women, who reported never using steroids, was of British standard in the Ms Figure category. Three women interviewed using the schedule reported using steroids. (One other female steroid-using bodybuilder talked to me but was loath to be formally interviewed.) Their usage, partly explicable in terms of their intimate relationships with male steroid-using bodybuilders, was largely a function of the 'type' of muscular body they wished to embody. The mean age of the interview sample was 30: a figure comparable to that noted by Pates and Barry (1996) in their survey of steroid users in South Wales. The oldest respondent to give their age was 53, the youngest 18. Only 16 per cent (N=11) stated they were 'officially' unemployed. Seven of these were weight trainers recruited in a prison, the remainder were bodybuilders, three of whom were receiving a regular income doing night club security work. There was a wide range of occupations, including: Youth and Community Worker, Fitness Instructor, Fire Fighter, Police Officer, Prosthetic Technician, Television Researcher. The majority of those officially employed were in skilled manual or clerical positions (Mechanic, Architectural Technician) and a few in the professions (Solicitor, Computer Programmer). These social demographics are comparable to those reported by Lenehan et al. (1996) in their survey of steroid users in the North West of England.

All the interviews were transcribed. The transcripts and ethnographic field notes were then indexed using computer coding software: 'Ethnograph' (Seidel and Clark 1984). Indexing of the field notes and transcripts has allowed a systematic approach to qualitative data analysis, helping to develop analytical propositions which apply to the entire universe of data carrying indexed codes. This approach is variously termed 'analytic induction' or 'deviant case analysis' (Bloor 1978).

Finally, an epistemological note. Adopting a position of 'subtle' as opposed to 'naïve' realism (Hammersley 1992), this book attempts to capture social complexity by developing theories grounded in data (Glaser and Strauss 1967). A correspondence theory of truth is retained which seeks to represent (not reproduce) reality (Hammersley 1992). In seeking to contribute knowledge that can be beneficial in expanding understanding, this study shares Miller and Glassner's

(1997) conviction that researchers may tap into, explore and learn about social realities existing outside of any particular interview situation engaged in by the researcher. Qualitative data may also be treated as a topic of analysis (Hammersley and Atkinson 1995: 126). Irrespective of the 'truth' or 'falsity' of what is said by the researched, participants draw from a (sub)cultural stock-of-knowledge to skilfully produce demonstrably 'morally adequate' accounts (Silverman 1993: 110). What may be particularly striking about data presented in this book, whether obtained through fieldwork or formally arranged depth interviews, is the amount of complex 'identity work' contained therein. Participants often know discrediting attributes are (stereo)typically associated with the category 'bodybuilder'. Displays of perspectives or moral forms (Silverman 1993), where narrators do 'being (extra)ordinary', are important considerations when reading extracts. Although the type of discourse analysis undertaken by some subcultural theorists (e.g. Widdicombe and Wooffitt 1995) is not attempted, the *functions* of members' accounts as 'situated narratives' are considered alongside their (possible) factual content.

Chapter outline

This chapter has provided a broad introduction. It defined the terms drug 'use' and 'abuse', reviewed some relevant literature, outlined the research, interview sample and epistemology. Chapter 2, the first empirical chapter, introduces the 'demonised' bodybuilding subculture. It describes orientations to lifting weights and bodybuilding, normalised instrumental drug use and bodybuilders' 'symbolic style' (Hebdige 1979). Chapter 3 identifies parameters for 'successful' bodybuilding: knowledge, dedication, finance and genetic potential. This subcultural system of relevances, instrumental in body- and identity-building, extends beyond 'risky' drug-taking patterns and behaviours (Augé and Augé 1999). Chapter 4 explores the spatially and temporally contingent task of creating 'the perfect body'. It questions critical feminist studies of bodybuilding and drug-taking, studies which label these 'risk' behaviours according to stereotyped constructs of personal inadequacy. Attention shifts in the next two chapters to bodybuilders' self-reflexively monitored use of physique-enhancing drugs. Focusing first upon the management of steroid risks, Chapter 5 describes bodybuilders' sophisticated ethnopharmacological knowledge and drug experimentation. Chapter 6 extends the analysis, detailing bodybuilders' knowledge and use of steroid accessory drugs and the subcultural exploration of competency, culpability and responsibility. Chapter 7, the final empirical chapter, explores bodybuilders' critical understandings of the 'Roid-Rage phenomenon. Chapter 8 concludes the book by underscoring the significance of preceding ethnographic observations in the social construction of 'appropriate' bodies and identities. It also underlines the rationale for bringing bodies back into social theory and identifies some possible policy implications vis-à-vis tertiary healthcare provision for steroid users.

Finally, it should be stressed that there are many different social scientific approaches to the study of the body, subjectivity, sport, gender and risk. While questioning some of these approaches, it is not a wholesale rejection of existing analytical traditions that leads me to follow a different approach, but a different set of analytic concerns. Using an empirically grounded approach, this book seeks to theorise bodybuilding and drug-taking as ongoing but variable practical accomplishments. Bringing lived bodies into social scientific studies is requisite for such purposes, serving both to question and complement existing academic work.

Chapter 2

Bodybuilding: a demonised drug subculture

Bodybuilding, similar to tattooing and scarification, has been associated with 'the improper, the dark side, the underworld, the demonic' (Young 1993: xx, cited by Pitts 1998: 70). Moreover, many bodybuilders qua reflexive body-subjects know, and can articulate upon the fact, that there exists a common negative reaction to them. One successful competitor remarked: 'People look at you as though you have two heads. You've got the comments, "he's a steroid freak, he's a steroid monster, uuggh, it looks sick, disgusting"' (Interview: Respondent 21). What may therefore seem puzzling is that 'bodybuilder' is not a given but a chosen identity, the result of individuals freely adopting to lead their lives (and construct their bodies) in particular ways. If elective bodybuilding 'spoils' the aesthetics, health and moral integrity of the embodied self then an obvious question presents itself: 'are bodybuilders irrational?'

Ethnographic research concerned with the nuances and social meanings of so-called 'deviancy' is often critical of the idea that such behaviour is symptomatic of an inadequate personality (e.g. Becker 1963, Taylor 1993). In sharing this conviction, the following endeavours to understand personal commitment to (chemical) bodybuilding by explicating members' routinised or commonsense understandings of social reality, their vocabulary of motives alongside their rational or calculative orientation to identified risk-behaviours. Centrally, it describes bodybuilders' subcultural understandings and background expectancies which enable them to rationalise and take-for-granted their everyday (deviant/dangerous/risky) activities.

Bodybuilding is first introduced by counterpoising mainstream with subcultural definitions. While some academic writings accurately define bodybuilding, what do members' accounts suggest about *outsiders'* interpretations, and how do participants describe bodybuilding from *their standpoint?* This strategy establishes bodybuilding as an exotic (or rather deviant) subculture, before using members' accounts to make familiar what is essentially foreign to a non-bodybuilding audience.

Orientations to lifting weights are then described. After first noting the (in)appropriateness of 'bodybuilding' and 'bodybuilder' as descriptive labels, the most readily identifiable features of bodybuilding are presented by contrasting the activity with weight-training and weight-lifting. Competition bodybuilding is then described alongside points of overlap with non-competition bodybuilding. This is necessary because both orientations promote an affinity to instrumental drug use. Gender issues are also broached, including qualifications to drug use and subcultural efforts to 'tame the beast in women's bodybuilding' (Bolin 1992a: 95). Bodybuilders' 'symbolic style' (Hebdige 1979) is then described before offering a closing statement on risk normalisation in a drug subculture.

Mainstream definitions and descriptions

Although 'bodies are in' (Frank 1990: 131) there is, even within today's fitness oriented cultural context, 'a residue of public disrespect still hovering over the bodybuilding community' (Klein 1993: 248). Ethnocentric descriptions of body-building, similar to Colonial misperception of native life, are identifiable within popular culture. For example, a literary critic, cited on the back cover of Fussell's (1991) bodybuilding narrative, describes the subculture as bizarre as any world found by Gulliver or Robinson Crusoe. Here bodybuilders, similar to 'risky' (delinquent) children who are cast as demons by adults (Scott *et al.* 1998: 696), are constructed as radically other. This separates them off from the 'real world' of those who have the power to define.

Bodybuilders contacted during this research, similar to British Bikers inter-viewed by McDonald-Walker (1998), frequently referred to the negatively-held prejudices in society deriving from popular conceptions of bodybuilders. Such imagery comes from a variety of sources, including the media, and frequently takes steroids and violence as definitive of bodybuilding and bodybuilding identity. Correspondingly, there is a general perception among bodybuilders that they inhabit a community under threat, leading many to engage in discursive stratagems to resist connotations of moral or social odium:

Zara, the gym orderly and steroid-using female bodybuilder, had *The Sunday Express* [British newspaper] which featured an article on steroids and bodybuilding [...] In the article was a short piece with a headline including terms such as 'Muscle Maniacs' and 'Irrational'. The article also discussed 'Roid-Rage. Bough read the article and became quite angry.

Bough: It pisses me off reading things like that. Fuck. If guys out there are acting like arseholes and are being aggressive, well it's an excuse. And for these papers to make out that we're all maniacs. That really gets on my nerves that does.

(Field Diary, 4 September 1994: Temple Gym)

Rod: Of course, you've got to live with the people around you who watch the news every night and whatever. But it's hard for them [the media] to say, to bring steroids out too openly and say: 'yes, if you do take them they're not going to make you blow a valve in your brain and throw a wobbly and a 'Roid-Rage'. But I think in one sense we shouldn't be victimised either by the public: 'oh my God, he's a bodybuilder, look at him, I bet he takes loads of them steroids and he's just waiting to flip any minute!' You know? We're not walking around like Rottweiler dogs. The image of bodybuilding is portrayed very poorly by the public in general really.

(Interview: Respondent 18)

Sociologists are also implicated in the articulation of these negative images. Concentrating upon the sport's elite, Klein (1993: 19) may offer the disclaimer that the bodybuilders depicted in his monograph are distillations exhibiting behaviour and attitudes more exaggerated than those of more moderate members of the bodybuilding community. Nevertheless, he dialectically draws from and reinforces unflattering stereotypes, thereby articulating a largely negative set of assumptions. Correspondingly, we are unable fully to appreciate the social construction of bodybuilding and associated 'risk' behaviours as 'normal', 'reasonable' and 'acceptable' for individuals routinely engaging in these activities. In endeavouring to understand bodybuilders' more favourable definition of the situation – and ultimately their commitment to the 'risky' practice of bodybuilding – the following humanises this demonised image.

)

Orientations to lifting weights

'Bodybuilder' and 'bodybuilding' as (in)appropriate labels

Describing various orientations to lifting weights, for the purposes of clearly demarcating bodybuilding subculture for analytic attention, would appear straightforward. However, classifying particular groups and subgroups – which, in an ethnography, necessitates close attention to participants' understandings – is not straightforward given the occasioned and contingent nature of 'lay' and sociological seeing (Silverman 1993: 201). The following statement was voiced by a young man who was loath to describe himself as a 'bodybuilder':

Barry: I know people who go for [bodybuilding] competitions but don't like to be classed as bodybuilders […] if a girl says: 'this is my boyfriend, he is a bodybuilder', there is a stigma attached to it. 'A bodybuilder, oh, steroids' and that type of thing, or 'he thinks he is hard' or something like that. Whereas if you say 'weight trainer' that has more to do with fitness which is more acceptable than just 'bodybuilder'.

(Interview: Respondent 44)

The usefulness of 'bodybuilder' as a membership categorisation device, representing a mode of conceptualisation for describing and explaining the empirical world, could be questioned. Certainly, affiliative members may resist category ascription; if bodybuilding is stigmatised then it may be situationally inappropriate for participants to openly embrace this identity. During everyday social interaction, information about the individual's 'real social identity' may remain undisclosed; in effect the 'bodybuilder' may conceal discrediting information about self for the purposes of 'passing' as normal (*cf.* Goffman 1968: 58).

There is also debate among bodybuilders concerning the inappropriateness of 'bodybuilding' as a descriptive label. Although calling themselves bodybuilders, several interviewees (including high-level competitors) favoured the term 'Physical Culture', and wanted participants to be called 'body-sculptors' not 'builders'. As suggested by Barry, the category-bound activity of drug-taking – 'risky' in the sense that it is stigmatised outside of bodybuilding subculture – partly explains this. Similar to adolescent Americans who may prefer to be called 'hotrodders' rather than 'teenagers', bodybuilders may favour alternative terms thus denying outsiders access to the known category-bound activities in which they may engage (Silverman 1993: 83).

In pointing to the deficiencies of 'bodybuilder' and 'bodybuilding' as descriptive labels, participants also stress their pursuit should be conceived as a process of shaping, refining and sculpting the body rather than simply building size. In asserting ownership of the descriptive apparatus, and in therefore attempting to assuage negative out-group assessments, bodybuilders emphasise the artistic features of their enterprise:

Mike: Bodybuilding is an unfortunate name for it. I'd like to see it more sort of ... I'd just like to see a nicer name for it. Bodybuilding's got a terrible sort of impression. Physical culture, something like that.

LM: That's what it was called in the past wasn't it?

Mike: Yeah, it would be a nicer term [...] body-sculpting. You know? More artistic.

(Interview: Respondent 15)

Furthermore, within the stratified bodybuilding subculture, divisions between participants in terms of competition status may mean there is variability in the application of the 'bodybuilder' label. In reporting social reality in all its complexity, it should be recognised that the meaning of this term is open to interpretation and is thus more or less relative. Nevertheless, as Mansfield and McGinn observe: 'a definitional structure exists in the sport [of bodybuilding] which powerfully influences what happens in the gym' (1993: 51). Consequently, it is possible to differentiate between various orientations to lifting weights in order to clarify what is distinct about being a 'bodybuilder' (which is itself a heterogeneous category) rather than a 'weight trainer' or 'weight lifter' (comprising of 'Olympic Weight-Lifting' and 'Power-Lifting').

The difference between weight-lifting, weight-training and bodybuilding

Bodybuilding may be distinguished from weight-lifting since the former activity takes as its goal improvement of physical appearance (bodily display), whereas the latter pursuit is aimed at lifting a maximum weight (bodily performance). On an analytic note, this cultivation of strength for displayed beauty (the bodybuilder's muscles) is suspect for non-participants because it is latently feminine, whereas beauty in the service of strength or courage (as among boxers, for example) is, by contrast, solidly masculine (Jefferson 1998: 84).

Weight lifters and bodybuilders train with weights, but neither category are 'weight trainers' as such. Weight trainers, who are typically fitness orientated and who possess a functionalist attitude towards the body, are described by Bednarek (1985: 241) in the following terms:

He [*sic*] has usually taken up weight-training to improve his physical fitness. This may be in the form of gaining strength in order to improve at his major sport, or to complement his aerobic training by anaerobic exercise. In general he is more concerned with losing weight or keeping his physique rather than gaining weight in terms of muscle growth.

Respondents also differentiated between various orientations to lifting weights. After asking 'what makes a weight trainer a bodybuilder?' one interviewee explained: 'the intention to improve the aesthetics of the physique rather than just to increase strength say, or fitness, or, fitness for a particular sport' (Interview: Respondent 25). Another bodybuilder, keen to present bodybuilding as a technically specialised pursuit, highlighted the differences between bodybuilding, weight-lifting (Olympic lifting) and weight-training. This excerpt also underscores the significance of bodybuilders' bodies as targets, which are constantly under surveillance and highly disciplined:

Carl: Well, bodybuilding you hit specific muscles and you train to build them like, your shoulders, traps [trapezius muscles located on the upper back], or whatever. With weight-lifting, you go to see what's the maximum that you can actually clean and jerk.

LM: That's like Olympic weight-lifting then?

Carl: It is Olympic weight-lifting.

LM: What about weight-training?

Carl: Well, weight-training I always class as people [...] who do it [training] once a week, this type of thing, that go down and lift a weight with no special motive. No co-ordination half of them. That's what I'd call weight-training. But bodybuilding is more scientific because you're setting out to alter the shape of your body, change your metabolism even. So it is a total difference.

(Interview: Respondent 33)

The different use of weights in bodybuilding and power-lifting (a non-Olympic sport requiring sheer strength as opposed to strength and agility) was also described by respondents. Again, this extract is noteworthy both as a source of information and a display of the narrator's positive self-conception:

Ken: Power lifter is completely different to a bodybuilder. As a power lifter they're trying to do one or two exercises with the maximum weight, and for a bodybuilder, like I say, I do sets [of exercises] of ten to fifteen [repetitions in contrast to the one repetition performed by power lifters].

BODYBUILDING: A DEMONISED DRUG SUBCULTURE

I'm shaping and sculpting my body. I'm more of an artist.

(Interview: Respondent 43)

Using contrast as a definitional strategy, one may outline the nature of body-building, describing what it is by highlighting what it is not. In contrast to various types of 'weight-lifting' (such as Olympic weight-lifting and power-lifting), body-builders are not preoccupied with bodily strength. Unlike fitness orientated 'weight trainers', bodybuilders (with the exception of Ms Figure-Fitness contenders discussed below) are concerned with radically changing their bodies. Rather than using weights in a casual fashion to tone their bodies, 'physique bodybuilders' commit themselves to specific and patterned training regimens in order to create what Mansfield and McGinn (1993: 51) term 'the outlandish body'.

Bodybuilders typically exercise in bodybuilding gyms rather than 'chromed up health spas' (Francis and Reynolds 1989: 23). Bodybuilding gyms therefore feature a concentration of this type of athlete. Some respondents, aware of the differential spatial distribution of types of people lifting weights, claimed a useful criterion for distinguishing bodybuilders from other categories of trainer is the type of gym which they frequent. Of course, social location shapes perception. Consequently, this rather generalised and inclusive view was more often expressed by contacts who mainly trained at home, leisure centres, or even a prison, rather than bodybuilding gyms. By exercising in a bodybuilding gym, divisions between gym members often become more visible to the observer.

Given the stigmatisation of bodybuilding, others attempted to normalise the activity by arguing that whether intentional or not, anybody and everybody who lifts weights is 'bodybuilding'. Bednarek (1985) similarly describes 'weight-training' for fitness as a type of bodybuilding. This encompassing view is under-standable because weight-training for whatever purpose (e.g. 'keeping-fit' and 'body-toning') invariably 'builds the body' to some extent. However, one may distinguish between physically doing 'bodybuilding' (specifically exercising and developing the body) and the generic social activity, consisting of formal organisations, rules and procedures, which is commonly known as 'bodybuilding'. One bodybuilder remarked: 'you are building your body [bodybuilding] when you're training, but when you actually compete, that's what bodybuilding is all about' (Interview: Respondent 9).

Performing bodybuilding type exercises may mean that somebody is doing 'bodybuilding' and there are people who consider themselves 'bodybuilders' by virtue of simply lifting weights in a bodybuilding gym. However, 'qualification' for group membership is dependent upon additional criteria. Indeed, for many competition orientated bodybuilders, the label 'bodybuilder' is only applicable to like minded gym members: 'other people are classed as weight trainers' (Interview:

31

Respondent 21). These (embodied) perceptions are, of course, spatially and temporally contingent. Within the stratified world of bodybuilding, differences between the categories 'bodybuilder' and 'weight trainer' are open to interpretation. A former competition bodybuilder commented:

Doug: I mean, if I was a competitive bodybuilder now, and you asked me [whether all people in the gym are bodybuilders] I would have said: 'no, only the competitive bodybuilders. All the others aren't'. You know what I mean? Like my answer would have been different. I mean, you must have heard people, you know, bodybuilders, competitive bodybuilders doing this and you'd say: 'do you think everyone in the gym is a bodybuilder?' And they'd say: 'no, just the bodybuilders, you know they're competitive and they belong to NABBA [National Amateur Body Building Association] or some other organisation and they're competing or have competed. All the rest aren't. They're just training'. It's a social thing with them isn't it? A bit of a pecking order, a bit of a structured thing, bodybuilding. Those at the top ... have you ever played golf? There's a bit of a hierarchy in golf as well. You know? The ones who are just learning, they're not really golfers at all. Although they think they are!

(Interview: Respondent 29)

Arguably, training with the intention of entering a competition is a strict definition of bodybuilding which is too exclusive (Mansfield and McGinn 1993: 51). Entering a bodybuilding show is a rite of passage clearly demarcating bodybuilders from other categories of weight trainer, but this is not a necessary qualification for group membership. Bodybuilding may be conceived as high in 'grid' (comprising of social distinctions and adherence to particular rules of conduct), but the strong 'group' boundary erected between participants and the outside world extends beyond formal competition status (cf. Douglas and Wildavsky 1982). The identification of bodybuilders is documented after delineating (non-)competition bodybuilding and establishing the 'normalised' but potentially risky use of physique-enhancing drugs.

(Non-)competition bodybuilding and 'normalised' drug use

Before describing the differences and similarities between competition and non-competition bodybuilding, and the subcultural acceptance of drug use, an important point requires emphasis. Namely, specific reference is made here to instrumental drug use for bodybuilding purposes. 'Recreational' drug-taking, where substances are taken as an end in themselves rather than a means to an end, provides a contrast to the ennobling and self-realising project of the dedicated drug-using bodybuilder (Bloor *et al*. 1998). Such activity was seldom reported or observed among bodybuilders (not weight trainers) contacted for this research. Certainly, recreational drug-taking may occur but the activity is widely considered inappropriate among those oriented and dedicated to (non-)competition bodybuilding.

Competition bodybuilding is geared towards entering an officially organised show. Hence, the label 'competition bodybuilder' is best regarded as a role individuals assume when preparing for, and competing in, physique or figure-fitness contests rather than a separate and distinct subtype of bodybuilder. These officially staged competitive events are organised by bodybuilding federations such as The National Amateur Body Building Association (NABBA), and the International Federation of Body Builders (IFBB). Competition bodybuilders are usually affiliated to one or more of these federations.

For many athletes the ethical value systems of their various sporting bodies prohibit drug-taking. Ban, which is a sign (objectivation) serving as a potent and explicit index of subjective meaning, casts an unmistakable shadow on the moral status of a particular act (Matza 1969: 146). Legislation against drug-taking therefore renders the activity morally guilty. However, if the 'authoritative' act of ban is either absent or systematically and openly flouted then the morality of drug use remains open. In Britain, only one bodybuilding federation (the Association of Natural Bodybuilders, abbreviated to ANB) promotes steroid-free competitions. Other federations do not test competitors for steroids and drug-taking is often deemed necessary among male and high level female physique competitors (Lowe 1998: 80).

Instrumental drug use is accepted and expected in men's physique competitions. A gym owner, for example, pointed to the marginal status of 'natural' competition bodybuilding as exemplified by the ANB and applauded the superior muscular development of drug assisted male athletes:

> You can see natural physiques on the beach, or on guys digging up the road. I mean, why go to see an ANB show when you can see a proper show instead? Who wants to see Mr. Steroid-free-pencil-neck when you can see Mr. Juggernaut?
>
> (Field Diary, 11 February 1996: Olympia Gym)

Gender as social practice that constantly refers to bodies and what bodies do (Connell 1995), requires emphasis when discussing the normalisation of drug use in competition bodybuilding. Similar to slip and kiln men working in pottery factories (Bellaby 1990), some male bodybuilders endeavoured, albeit in slick and subtle ways, to maintain sharp group (and bodily) boundaries by excluding women. One strategy was the disapprobation of testosterone use by female bodybuilders. An elite male bodybuilder, after saying 'it doesn't make sense to me for a woman to take testosterone. If I had to take oestrogen to compete in the Olympia [high level professional competition] I'd be out of there', added:

> As a man it seems OK, quite logical to take more testosterone … but for a woman! Besides, that look [Ms Physique] is going out. You've got the Ms Fitness coming in – a shape that is seen as more pleasing to both men and women. There's no pressure for women to take testosterone. That look is being replaced.
>
> (Field Diary, 3 April 1995: Seminar by professional bodybuilder)

To slightly modify the above remark, within and without bodybuilding subculture there is considerable 'pressure for women *not* to take testosterone'. Here, constraints apply to women's means (bodybuilding technologies) as well as their ends (muscular body). This point, concordant with a phenomenological approach to risk (Bloor 1995: 98), may also be subjected to an explicitly cultural theorisation. The differential treatment of the sexes in bodybuilding, similar to boxing, 'provides an example of the way in which biological arguments have been applied systematically to women's bodies in order to control cultural practices' (Hargreaves 1997: 38).

Both male and female physique bodybuilders – rather than Ms Figure-Fitness competitors who are a 'toned down' version of the physique category (St Martin and Gavey 1996: 48) – usually exhibit substantial muscularity. These '*gains*' are usually achieved through several years of training, dieting and drug-taking. (Sub)cultural disparagement notwithstanding, instrumental drug use among high level female bodybuilders is concordant with the hierarchist orientation to risk (high grid and high group) where risk behaviour may be high in close conformity with prevailing group norms (*cf.* Bloor 1995: 94). As remarked by a non-steroid-using female physique competitor who was successful in Wales but who was overshadowed by the level of muscularity displayed by Ms Physique bodybuilders at the NABBA Britain line-up:

Julie: You'd be better off taking something [bodybuilding drugs] if you want to get to the top as that's the only way you're going to do it [...] OK, you can win [a national title in Wales] and not take the stuff, but if they [body-building federations] want big, huge physiques that are ripped to the bone with cuts and veins [i.e. displaying virtually no body-fat], then the only way you're going to get that is through taking artificial substances. I mean, you can't do that naturally, your body is just not capable of producing that kind of physique.

(Interview: Respondent 11)

Ms Figure-Fitness competitors, who have now 'eclipsed' Ms Physique body-builders in popularity, also enter bodybuilding shows and are evaluated according to body aesthetics. However, these competitors retain a beauty-pageant level of feminine presentation (St Martin and Gavey 1996: 48), typically providing a side show for male bodybuilders. In displaying lower levels of muscularity these women are less likely to take steroids but other drugs such as Clenbuterol and Tamoxifen may assist pre-contest preparation (see Chapter 6). These women are generally welcomed at bodybuilding competitions. Similar to women who are accoutrements to male boxing, Ms Figure-Fitness bodybuilders 'are "displayed" as stereotyped, (hetero)sexualized commodities in swimsuits [and] high-heeled shoes' (Hargreaves 1997: 47).

Before entering a show both male and female bodybuilders must adhere to a calorie reduced diet for approximately twelve weeks in order to get into 'competition shape' – a transitory state rarely lasting more than a few days. This entails 'cutting up' and for the Physique class 'getting ripped' (achieving an extremely low level of body-fat). Diminishing subcutaneous body-fat is necessary in order clearly to show one's muscular development to the scrutinising eyes of the judges, the audience and, perhaps most importantly, oneself. This latter point concerning the body as an object for critical self-appraisal should be stressed. The volitional act of entering a bodybuilding competition is dependent upon the individual's desire to appropriate, control and assert ownership over the material body. This rationalised goal, explicit in bodybuilding and a feature of sport in general (Cashmore 1998: 84), is shared by all fe/male muscle enthusiasts and is a basis of commonality for (non-)competition 'bodybuilders'.

Bodybuilding may, in accord with the ascetic Protestant ethic, represent the rationalisation and regulation of the human body but countervailing baroque and postmodern tendencies are evidenced. For example, the public spectacle of the bodybuilding show, similar to the burlesque ballet in seventeenth-century baroque culture, opens up the possibility of the feminisation of male 'dancers' and the representation of grotesque bodies (Turner 1996: 16). Oiled, shaved and tanned to enhance the visibility of their muscles, competition bodybuilders display their sculpted bodies to a judging panel in front of an audience and receive feedback on how 'good' they are in comparison to others (Bednarek 1985: 240). As ceremonial acts comparable to traditional rites of passage, bodybuilding competitions draw much of their meaning from the presence of the audience (*cf.* Klesse 1999: 22).

Judging criteria, especially in female physique bodybuilding, are frequently contested, are a source of controversy and are dynamic (Guthrie and Castelnuovo 1992). However, among conflicting views there is overlap and consensus. Somatic criteria relate to the proportions and harmony of the physique (*'symmetry'*), muscle form, size and definition (Lowe 1998). A look of proportionate balance is perhaps of central significance:

> Symmetry is regarded as one of the primary characteristics that judges look for in a contest. It is not so much of a factor as to who has the biggest body parts, but rather how these parts blend together.
>
> (Thirer and Greer 1978: 197)

Competition bodybuilders, described as choreographers by one interviewee, must present their bodies correctly; the ability to pose being essential (Thirer and Greer 1978: 187). In the physique classes posing entails standing on stage next to other competitors while performing '*mandatories*' (compulsory poses) such as '*front and rear double biceps*', '*lat-spread*', '*abs*' and '*side triceps*'. Ms Figure-Fitness competitors also perform bodybuilding poses, but certain poses are omitted. This may be considered part of the process where 'transgressive' female bodybuilding is rendered 'safe' to the gender order. In the male controlled bodybuilding subculture 'appropriately' female bodies and identities are constructed and performed:

Monique: Then there is your bikini round – which is your bodybuilding round – where you do compulsory poses. But what they're doing is taking out a lot of the poses that are akin to bodybuilding. So, for instance, we are only doing double biceps from the front, rear double biceps and chest – that's all we're doing. We're not doing abs [abdominal muscles], we're not doing lat-spread, we're not doing triceps. None of that.

LM: Is that because bodybuilding for females is considered a bit too masculine?

Monique: Masculine, yeah. So they wanna do away with that.

(Interview: Respondent 12)

After being judged together each bodybuilder then performs an individualised posing routine to a piece of music of their choice. These choices often enhance and display the competitors' gender; for example, 'seductive' versus 'power poses' and love songs versus rock music (Lowe 1998: 122–3). Individual posing routines are followed by a '*pose down*' where all competitors in a particular height, weight, age, or experience category collectively perform free-style poses to music.

Entering a bodybuilding competition is unimportant for male '*power bodybuilders*' and '*smooth mass monsters*' (bodybuilders striving for strength and size without wishing to reduce calories). Similarly, competitions are inconsequential to bodybuilders who are 'not really into that ballet shit' (Interview: Respondent 24), those who lack financial resources (contest preparation is expensive – see Chapter 3), prefer to cultivate a 'body beautiful' as opposed to a 'body freak' (see Chapter 4), are at the early stages of their bodybuilding career, or who are generally unwilling and/or unable to commit themselves to the extremely ascetic dietary, training and drug regimens strictly adhered to by most competition bodybuilders.

In short, while enhancing bodily aesthetics is a goal similarly shared by those assuming the role of the non-competition bodybuilder, in contrast to their competition orientated gym mates they have little ambition to participate in bodybuilding shows. However, in discussing the similarities between competition and non-competition bodybuilding, and in highlighting the 'normalised' practice of instrumental drug use among various strata of bodybuilder, it should be recognised that all participants place a premium on enhancing bodily aesthetics. Irrespective of the 'demands' of formal competitions, all bodybuilders may therefore be described as competitive: ongoing bodily development is a physically arduous process entailing a struggle against the dictates of nature. Certain pharmaceuticals are instrumental in this process; hence, an affinity also exists between (non-)competition bodybuilding and drug use.

To be sure, instrumental drug use may be inconsequential to participants because of limited interest or 'motivational relevances' (Bloor 1995: 98). Not all bodybuilders (regularly) use physique-enhancing drugs. Bodybuilders have various different and overlapping reasons for rejecting or limiting their personal drug use. The varying ways in which bodybuilders orient to steroids and analogous drugs may be considered a product of cultural variation (Douglas 1985), or, more dynamically, shifting 'systems of relevances' (Schutz 1970):

If concern about drug side effects is topically and motivationally relevant then 'barriers' to drug-taking, similar to the ethic of sexual restraint in the time of HIV/AIDS (Lupton and Tulloch 1998), may be phrased in terms of the care of the self in an environment of risk. For example, bodybuilders adopting an 'egalitarian' orientation to risk during an ethnographic interview, and who thus view the naturalistic body as ephemeral/fragile/precarious (Adams 1995: 40), cite possible and/or actual health problems. The female body, for wholly social reasons, is deemed especially vulnerable to steroids given irreversible and highly visible virilising 'side effects' such as facial hair. Such effects are likely to *remain* problematic (embarrassing) for many women because of volitional ('intrinsic') and other-constrained ('imposed') topical relevances (Bloor 1995: 98). Self-other bodily evaluations are significant because bodybuilders' identities are crucially shaped by their physical appearance in a (sub)culture where Cooley's 'looking glass self' (1983) is no longer a mere metaphor.

Other relevances shaping and constraining instrumental drug use include: finance and possessing favourable genetics for accruing muscle (see Chapter 3), variable body-projects (see Chapters 4 and 5), and personal satisfaction derived from accruing muscle 'naturally'. The modern pristine body is associated with naturalness (Pitts 1998: 70), and many bodybuilders state they are 'natural' (steroid free) despite consuming other 'technologies of the self' including supplements and past steroid use. Unsurprisingly, invocation of the 'natural' is often salient among women bodybuilders who 'are considered transgressive of the natural order of things' (Balsamo 1995: 217). Finally, the possibility of legal sanctions in certain countries, but not in South Wales during this study, may regulate drug-taking. Taking chemically and symbolically 'impure' substances – irrespective of the subcultural acceptance of instrumental drug use – may therefore be rejected or limited by fe/male bodybuilders through fear of spoiling the integrity of the body and identity (Goffman 1968).

Physique-enhancing drugs may be avoided. However, from contacts established with a wide range of bodybuilders, this research found that many participants (including ANB competitors) have used physique-enhancing drugs. Furthermore, similar to ethnographic studies of intravenous drug-injecting (McKeganey 1990), I found that drugs were spoken about in a matter-of-fact way:

> Andrew had just finished telling me about his attempts to increase the size of his arms by injecting Sustanon 250 and Deca [types of steroid] directly into his biceps. He claimed a professional bodybuilder, famous for his tricep development, used the same technique. Jimmy, who had recently competed in the Mr. Wales, and who had regained some 'mass' after ceasing his calorie reduced diet, then walked over. Tongue in cheek, Andrew exclaimed: 'Here's fat boy!' Jimmy, taking the comment in good humour, replied: 'Nah, I shouldn't get too fat. I'm taking Spiro' [Spiropent or Clenbuterol]. Andrew mimicked the hand tremors which sometimes accompany Clenbuterol usage, adding: 'If I take four in the morning, I'm like that'. Billy, a gym instructor who was also nearby, quipped: 'Well, you'd have no need for a food blender for your protein shakes then'.
>
> (Field Diary, 27 May 1999: Adonis Gym)

Even among those bodybuilders who said that they personally had never used steroids, there seemed to be widespread acceptance that drugs were a part of their world. However, bodybuilders expressing pro-drug attitudes generally qualified their statements; in adopting the hierarchist orientation to risk onus was placed upon 'proper' management (Adams 1995). For example, steroids were only considered 'all right' in moderation (see Chapters 5 and 7). A bodybuilder, who had competed with the ANB and who claimed to have never used steroids, said:

Frank: I personally got nothing against steroids because I know, if they're used and not abused, then they can be a good thing rather than a bad thing [...] if it's used in the right quantities ... I don't think there's anything wrong with it.

(Interview: Respondent 41)

In addition, steroids were only considered appropriate if the user observes parameters for successful bodybuilding (see Chapter 3), specific substances were considered illegitimate bodybuilding drugs (see Chapter 6), and it was widely accepted that ANB competitors should be 'drug-free' (though the precise meaning of this term was open to interpretation). Finally, some bodybuilders felt teenagers should avoid steroids given the risk of premature physeal closure and the stunting of growth (cf. American Academy of Pediatrics 1997: 905–6):

Bill: I don't like to see kids under sort of – I say under 20, but there's lots of people under that age using steroids now. I would say now, realistically, I would say 16 to 18 [is the youngest to be using steroids]. And I don't like saying it but, you know? If I was the absolute ruler of it all I would say 20/ 21 before you even touch your first steroids. Maybe even 25 because you're still growing ... the bone ends and things. It causes premature closing of the bone ends if you're not careful.

(Interview: Respondent 24)

In sum, bodybuilding may be conceived as a variegated and stratified world. For example, there are differences between competition and non-competition bodybuilding, natural and non-drug tested competitions, and types of competitor (e.g. Physique and Figure-Fitness). Drug use may therefore be considered more or less appropriate depending upon various orientations to bodybuilding. Nevertheless, bodybuilders' shared goal of 'enhancing' physical appearance results in a shift in conception so that drug use is a conceivable possibility for all participants. This, alongside the everyday taken-for-granted nature of drug use, renders drug-taking (or more specifically, the instrumental use of physique-enhancing drugs) a normalised practice among bodybuilders.

BODYBUILDING, DRUGS AND RISK

Identifying bodybuilders

The identification of bodybuilders, similar to the identification of the Lue in Thailand (*cf.* Silverman 1993: 54–5), is clearly dependent upon their successful presentation of themselves as a collectivity. And, if bodybuilding is something of a demonised subculture, there may be good reasons why the identification 'bodybuilder' is avoided in everyday life. However, if bodybuilders are conceived as a social group existing in the empirical world, then members' accounts are a useful resource for identifying individuals comprising the bodybuilding collectivity.

Identity symbols in the form of embodied signs, which convey social information and which establish group membership, have been noted by various sociologists and anthropologists (e.g. Brain 1979, Goffman 1968). Visual indices, and auditory indices in the form of speech, signify affiliation to bodybuilding subculture. Importantly, embodied signs represent indigenous criteria for identifying 'bodybuilders', distinguishing 'insiders' from 'outsiders' (including 'marginal members' such as weight trainers). The criteria for identification of bodybuilding identity, which relate to bodybuilders' symbolic style, are noted below.

The symbolic use of style, signifying membership in a particular role, is a well documented theme in subcultural analyses. According to Hebdige (1979), the expressive forms and mundane objects of such diverse groups as Punks, Rastafarians and Mods possess a symbolic dimension and are signs of identity. Dreadlocks, safety pins, pointed shoes and scooters are meaningful objects which denote, among other things, affiliation to a particular subculture (Hebdige 1979: 2–3). Certainly, and in following Sweetman (1999: 66), more contemporary forms of body modification such as tattooing and piercing 'appear to act less as markers of group identification, and more as markers of the self'. This argument about 'expressive individualism' correlates well with the claim that bodybuilding is a reflexive project of the self. However, the importance of style in expressing commitment to a *specific* subculture – the bodybuilding collectivity – was commented upon by some:

Jack: You can tell a weight trainer from a bodybuilder in the gym like. You know? You can see the difference. They'll buy [nutritional] supplements, they'll wear the clothes, it's a whole lifestyle. They'll go to the shows [competitions]. Some people [weight trainers] just move the weights.

(Interview extract: Respondent 10)

Following Jack's observation, it is clear that various criteria, extending beyond formal competition status, are used by bodybuilders to identify other subcultural

40

members. Indeed, while group affinity based upon heterogeneity is evidenced among 'bodybuilders' (see Chapter 4), this 'alliance' is well defined, allowing sociological discussion of 'subcultural' criteria. Bodybuilders' subcultural style may be subjected to focused consideration, where membership is signified by the actor's image, demeanour and argot (Brake 1980: 12), alongside the individual's degree of commitment to bodybuilding as a radical 'lifestyle choice' (Giddens 1991).

'Image' refers to appearance, composed of costume, accessories such as hairstyle, jewellery and artefacts (Brake 1980: 12). For bodybuilders, regular training sessions and frequent showers render short haircuts practical. However, because hairstyles are gendered displays, most male bodybuilders sport short haircuts while female bodybuilders often have long (blonde) hair (Lowe 1998: 123–4). Clothes are also relevant. Using the comparative method favoured by social anthropologists, a former bodybuilder writes (Fussell 1991: 131):

> Our home was like a sumo wrestler's stable. In place of the mawashi (the ceremonial diaper), the geta (wooden sandals), and the formal kimona worn by the sumotori outside the stable, we wrapped ourselves in our layers of Gold's Gym clothes. They defined who we were and what we did.

Furthermore, physical appearance or 'body-image' may be added to Brake's (1980: 12) list when discussing 'image' as a component of subcultural style. For bodybuilders, the appropriate look comprises of '*size*' (enlarged musculature) which is also '*defined*' (clearly visible):

John: Just 'cause you had big arms, big shoulders but a big fat gut, you wouldn't be classed as a bodybuilder. You'd just be classed as like someone who lifts weights, just works-out. But unless you got that look about you like … if you're in good shape or whatever, yeah, you'd be classed as a bodybuilder like.

(Interview: Respondent 35)

Bodybuilders also have a special argot or vocabulary. As noted by Klein (1993: 30): 'terms such as abs, delts, cuts, gains, presses, 'roids [...] and bitch-tits are likely to evoke an emotional response from these people as the notion of trickle-down economics would to a Reagan loyalist'. Bodybuilders' shared argot is most clearly evidenced when talking about steroid use (see Chapter 5).

'Demeanour', which is made up of expression, gait and posture, is an additional element of style (Brake 1980: 12). A well documented aspect of male bodybuilders' demeanour is their style of walking: something which may be considered integral in the construction of masculine identity (Jefferson 1998: 78) but which has also been compared to the performance of emphasised femininity (Fussell 1994: 45). Elsewhere Fussell states that 'The Walk' is a 'not-so-secret signal among the iron cognoscenti of the presence of a dues-paying member of the bodybuilding guild' (1991: 54). Fussell describes 'The Walk', as performed by his two gym mates:

> I watched as [they] strutted down the street. They swept their arms out to the side, as if the sheer massivity of their lat wings necessitated it. They burrowed their heads slightly into their shoulders to make their necks appear larger. They looked bowlegged, absurdly stiff, and infinitely menacing.
>
> (Fussell 1991: 54–5)

The 'natural' act of walking often functions as a communicational code and is a result of applied body-techniques of socialisation (Falk 1995: 95–6). Fussell (1991), similar to Maori girls who are urged by their mothers to adopt the 'right' gait (Mauss 1973: 74), was taught the walk of the bodybuilder by his two new gym mates. However, although 'The Walk' is communicative, its subcultural legitimacy is dependant upon muscle acquisition. Neophytes, for example, risk being ridiculed by other gym members if they walk this way: 'Aghh, look at him! He's got ILS [Imaginary Lat Syndrome]'. Moreover, 'Kiting' (looking like a kite) or 'Carpet Carrying' (appearing to be carrying two invisible roles of carpet parallel under the arms), draws negative attention to the subculture irrespective of bodily capital. Some narrators reflected upon this at a time when bodybuilding was increasingly being stigmatised:

Len: Yeah and with the size often comes a certain swagger. They walk very cocky. They walk into a place and you can tell straight away they're full of themself. And because you're a big built lad you haven't got to thrust your arms out at a forty-five degree angle and walk like you just shit yourself. You've got so many guys walking around like that and it makes us all look an idiot. Because that's the archetypal or whatever the word is, the walk of the bodybuilder. Everybody says: 'oh, you do weights do you?' And they go into this silly little strut, arms out at forty-five degrees. Well, I don't fucking walk like that and I'm 18 stone so, why these like little like 14-stone lads do it I really don't understand. Trying to make themselves look bigger than they are.

(Interview: Respondent 23)

Image, argot and demeanour may be important components in signifying group membership. However, perhaps of most importance is the extent to which the individual adheres to the bodybuilding principles of training, nutrition and recuperation (see Chapter 3). As stated by one bodybuilder: 'a weight trainer becomes a bodybuilder when he does it [training] seriously, say three times a week or four times a week, and he's focused on his training, eating and sleeping' (Interview: Respondent 8). In short, bodybuilders immerse themselves in a certain mode-of-being, and commit themselves to bodybuilding regimens which, in Giddens' (1991) sense, represent a 'radical lifestyle choice'. Although competitions demand strict adherence to bodybuilding principles, being a bodybuilder apparently has less to do with entering a physique competition, and more to do with embracing the daily ascetic regimes which characterise the everyday life world of bodybuilding. Correspondingly, bodybuilding, like sea diving, 'is not simply a hobby but a way of life which defines moral worth and identity' (Hunt 1995: 442).

It is here, perhaps, that bodybuilders may be compared to various religious groups who set themselves apart by their food, clothes and general lifestyle. For example, members of the Hare Krishna cult or the Old-Order Amish of Pennsylvania, USA, are extreme examples of the successful use of styles in maintaining a unique way of life (Brain 1979: 154–5). Such groups are also implicated in the culture of risk where internal hardship is a source of inner strength, offering resistance to pollution of their ways of life from without (Bellaby 1990: 471).

The specifics of bodybuilding as a radical lifestyle choice – the significance of training, nutrition and recuperation in the construction of 'appropriate' bodies and identities – are explored in the next chapter. However, the argument that bodybuilding is a distinct lifestyle is mentioned here in order to highlight the difference between various orientations to lifting weights. Irrespective of competition status, individuals are generally considered 'bodybuilders' if they look, dress, act and talk a certain way. Certainly, as a stratified world comprising of participants who are competition and non-competition orientated, variability exists in the application of the 'bodybuilder' label. The successful identification of bodybuilders is further confounded if participants, through fear of stigmatisation, conceal their group affiliation. Nevertheless, despite difference and contingency there are important points of overlap and constancy.

Conclusion

Focusing upon deep sea divers' normalisation of risk, Hunt (1995: 441) states that 'normal risk' entails 'practices that specific persons on specific occasions formulate as necessary, appropriate, reasonable or understandable'. Within the demonised bodybuilding subculture, self-identified bodybuilders (and other affiliative members) whom I talked with and observed in daily life, constructed instrumental drug use as a legitimate means for attaining a subculturally prescribed goal. To be sure, personal usage may be limited or rejected for various reasons; for example, gendered discourses and the invocation of the 'natural' constrain female bodybuilding practices. Also, concerns about being discredited outside of the subculture may be topically relevant resulting in bodybuilders disavowing what non-members (and 'marginal members' such as weight trainers) consider 'unacceptable' risk-inducing behaviour. Although qualified, the pro-drug attitudes reported above were expressed by a range of bodybuilders during fieldwork and depth interviews. These shared understandings, acquired by participants within the bodybuilding *habitus*, contribute to the sustainability of chemical bodybuilding as an ongoing practical accomplishment.

The subcultural normalisation of 'risk' also extends beyond (mostly male) bodybuilders' instrumental drug-taking activities. As noted, bodybuilders, although perhaps expressing reservations about the appropriateness of the 'bodybuilder' label through fear of spoiling the social self (Goffman 1968), are well motivated to present their sport and/or art in a positive light. Such rhetorical appeals, in assuaging common negative perceptions of bodybuilding identity and activities, are ideologically supportive. Individuals embracing bodybuilding, who are identifiable through their 'symbolic style' and commitment to bodybuilding as a radical 'lifestyle choice', are able (though perhaps not necessarily willing in certain interactional contexts) to negotiate definitions of risk which support the fundamental tenets of their drug subculture. Carefully planned drug use (not abuse) among competent bodybuilders is deemed instrumental in creating and recreating types of 'perfect' muscular body. In accord with the hierarchist orientation to risk and risk management (*cf.* Adams 1995), these pro-drug attitudes are generally qualified in terms of gender and age considerations.

The craving for success in sport has been linked to risk behaviours, including drug-taking (Blake 1996: 150). The next chapter identifies parameters for 'successful' bodybuilding: parameters which incorporate, but which also extend beyond, drug use. This provides a contrast to recent studies which claim bodybuilders' 'risky' drug use patterns and behaviours create 'successful' training programmes (Augé and Augé 1999: 217).

Chapter 3

Parameters for successful bodybuilding

Clinicians have claimed multiple drug use patterns create 'successful' bodybuilding training programmes, rendering bodybuilders at significant risk for use (Augé and Augé 1999: 217). However, the imposed risk of social stigmatisation, rather than the intrinsic risk of self-administering potentially harmful drugs, may be more topically relevant for bodybuilders:

> ... we have to beat this drug rap that it [bodybuilding] has. That's one of the most unfortunate things. I'm not crazy about people knowing I'm a bodybuilder because one of the questions I get asked right away is, 'What about steroids? Do you use steroids?' On and on ... They think that's all bodybuilding is.
>
> (Zane 1997: 62)

In a culture where claiming personal responsibility for health becomes an exercise in personal virtue (Frank 1997: 105), illicit drug-taking represents a deviation from righteous living. Correspondingly, in the social construction of 'appropriate' bodies and identities, bodybuilding success cannot simply be attributed to drug use irrespective of the symbolic centrality and instrumental capacity of various physique-enhancing substances.

Experienced bodybuilders claim success is dependent upon many factors (Thirer and Greer 1978: 187). These factors may be subsumed under a four part typology, representing an 'ideal typical' construct (Weber 1976) which is embodied in its purity only among stylised bodybuilders and which incorporates a system of relevances accepted beyond question by the in-group. Importantly, these typifications constitute the general framework of the cultural setting pregiven to single actors as a scheme of orientation and interpretation of their actions (Schutz 1964: 252). Immersion in bodybuilding, an awareness of the subjective meaning of the group, indicates ongoing muscular development is more or less dependent upon:

- Knowledge (of training, nutrition and drugs).
- Dedication (commitment to an ascetic lifestyle).
- Finance (bodybuilding can prove expensive), and
- Genetics (natural bodily potential).

This typology, concordant with Wacquant's (1995a: 70) observation that the 'flexible' body may be significantly restructured within given parameters, identifies several diverse aspects incorporating various dimensions. These relevances are instrumental to bodybuilders in two main ways. They are prescriptions and conditions for success – which, incidentally, may be considered postmodern because they frame men's *and* women's bodybuilding activities (*cf.* Glassner 1990) – and they constitute an ideological reserve. Bodybuilders' identities may be at risk but participants are able to draw upon this system and integrate it into their self-definition. Here bodybuilding is both an aesthetic project of the self and a means of constructing subjectivity (Lupton 1997: 143).

This chapter documents the subcultural significance of these four parameters for body- and identity-building. Similar to the previous chapter, the perceived athletic, artistic and scientific features of bodybuilding are reported. The extent to which bodybuilding is a radical 'lifestyle choice' (Giddens 1991) is also explored further. Training, nutrition, and drug-taking are briefly considered in relation to 'knowledge'. However, ethnopharmacological knowledge is detailed in Chapters 5 and 6.

Finally, it should be recognised that bodybuilding 'success' may be analysed from various angles. There are, for instance, important issues concerning the interplay of economic, ideological and political forces which define types of gendered muscular body that are marketable and are thus rewarded (Lowe 1998). Moreover, the social activity of bodybuilding – while bounded and comprising identifiable rules of conduct – is highly individualised. Correspondingly, and as will be elaborated in the next chapter, creating 'the perfect body' is a variable project. Nevertheless, the four parameters detailed below provide a framework for creating championship standard bodies. In this chapter 'success' is therefore defined as the ability to create these subculturally valorised bodies which are muscular, symmetrical and low-fat.

Knowledge

Within popular discourse one may identify the 'Law of Compensation, which postulates an inverse relationship between mind and muscle, between athletic and intellectual development' (Cashmore 1998: 87). Unsurprisingly, many bodybuilders are critical of this argument, claiming there is instead a proportionate relationship between mind and muscle. Bodybuilding success, it is argued, presupposes knowledge. This claim is thoroughly grounded in the lived realities of their enterprise.

In highlighting the significance of knowledge in successful bodybuilding, reference is not being made to bodybuilders' powers of abstract thought. Rather, in following Schutz's (1964) work on the phenomenology of knowledge, it is being suggested that bodybuilding success (especially at the national level of competition and beyond) is dependent upon clear and distinct understanding based on information rather than mere sentiment. Many bodybuilders endorse the view that theirs is a knowledge-empowered community, and that accruing knowledge is instrumental in accruing muscle. A former professional world champion said: 'Bodybuilders sometimes have this reputation for being big stupid guys, muscle-heads, but it's literally impossible to be like that and be a top pro. You need a vast knowledge of nutrition and training' (Yates 1994: 92).

A detailed and technically sophisticated (ethno)scientific stock-of-knowledge is identifiable within bodybuilding subculture. This knowledge is derived from various sources, including medicine which is neither fully accepted nor rejected by information-seeking bodybuilders (Monaghan 1999b). Knowledge and competency in bodybuilding also presupposes learning through habit and exercise (Bourdieu et al. 1991). Comparable with neophytes to marihuana (Becker 1963), novice bodybuilders must 'learn the techniques'.

While bodybuilding may be considered a drug-subculture, Becker's (1963) model describing the career of the drug taker could be applied to several aspects of the muscle-building enterprise. Bodybuilding success is not simply a function of learning the (complex) drug-taking techniques necessary for entering into a regularised and systematic pattern of drug use. Learning about supplements, exercise and nutrition is also important (Phillips 1996: 11).

Knowledge in bodybuilding delineates and defines normative action, serving as a *guideline* for individual practice. This generalised knowledge is extremely flexible and must ultimately be individually tailored. Similar to the pluralism of the medieval Church, there is a multiplicity of forms of 'bodybuilding' to the extent that bodybuilding, like Catholicism, is capable of incorporating into itself 'a repertoire of inherited and shared beliefs and symbols, [which remain] capable of enormous flexibility' (Duffy 1992: 3, cited by Mellor and Shilling 1997: 69). Personal experimentation therefore crucially shapes various aspects of body-builders' shared knowledge, including knowledge of:

- *Drug Use*: 'Ethnopharmacological' knowledge concerning types of drugs, length of time on drugs and the time off between courses, reasons for varying drug dosages, using different drugs simultaneously and sequentially.
- *Training and Recuperation*: 'Ethnophysiological' knowledge, including an understanding of the various muscle groups which should be trained, appropriate exercises for stimulating muscular hypertrophy, time needed for muscles to recover.
- *Diet and Nutritional Supplementation*: 'Ethnonutritional' knowledge concerning the 'correct' amount of macro-nutrients – protein, complex carbohydrates, fat – in the diet. Knowledge of pre-contest dietary techniques and the timing of meals. Understanding the (limited) role of nutritional supplements.

Because bodybuilding ethnopharmacology is explored later in the book, this section only reviews points two and three. First, however, various sources of information are noted.

Sources of information in bodybuilding

According to Giddens (1991: 194), 'in conditions of high modernity, in many areas of social life – including the domain of the self – there are no determinant authorities'. In such a context of pluralism, information may be gleaned from various sources by individuals wishing to (chemically) construct the physical (and social) self. As stated by Nettleton and Watson (1998: 6): 'The reflexive self is one which relies on a vast array of advice and information provided in a myriad of sources'.

Knowledge in bodybuilding, although partly derived from an individual's own accumulated and experimental body of experience, is also obtained through face-to-face interaction with more experienced members. For instance, seasoned competition bodybuilders are usually helpful in advising others with aspirations to compete. Gym owners, who often have experience as competition bodybuilders, are also a source of knowledge (Korkia and Stimson 1993: 122–3). Importantly, knowledge frames men's and women's bodybuilding but the imparting and acquisition of certain knowledges is gendered. For example, it is mostly practising male bodybuilders who socialise women competitors by acting as mentors (Lowe 1998: 29). No doubt, such processes support heterosexual imperatives – the socially prescribed need for women to be attractive and to please men.

Technical information on the intricacies of bodybuilding is also readily obtained through various global media of communication including booklets, magazines and, more recently, the Internet. Literary sources of information – what Giddens (1991) would term 'guides to living' – are usually written by male bodybuilders specifically for a fe/male bodybuilding audience. This empirical observation aligns with feminist criticism of scientific discourse where women are less involved in the production of science as a form of cultural activity (cf. Watson 2000: 49–50). Bodybuilders' (ethno)scientific genderised texts include 'chemical' guides to living such as 'steroid handbooks' (e.g. Duchaine 1989, Phillips 1991). Most steroid users, in making a 'religion' out of rationality, are 'avid consumers of information about AS [steroids]' (Korkia and Stimson 1993: 123). There is, of course, a temporal dimension to this and changing zones of relevance which reflect fluctuating 'interests at hand' (Schutz 1970). Subcultural pharmacopoeia are typically consumed more avidly at certain critical junctures; for example, when the decision is first made to use physique-enhancing drugs, or experiment with a 'new' drug or combination of drugs. Here 'risk' information is actively sought during 'fateful moments' which are potentially damaging to the protective cocoon which defends ontological security (Giddens 1991: 114).

Doubt about the validity of all knowledges means that various sources of 'expertise' may be incorporated into subcultural and individual knowledge systems. There is within bodybuilding a complex intermixing of lay beliefs and scientific knowledge, representing the dialectic of social and scientific rationality in 'risk society' (Beck 1992, Williams and Bendelow 1998). In the quest for physical perfection, and in surveying possible risks associated with drug use, bodybuilders claim any and all information (including medical knowledge) may be relevant (Phillips 1991: 9). This supports Lupton and Tulloch's (1998: 19) argument that the 'unfinished' projects of the body and the self often require individuals to make use of expert knowledges, particularly those of medicine. Certainly, body-building is heavily inflected with the discourse of science (Schulze 1990: 69); this is permissible because knowledge is literally translated into physical power and thus muscle growth. An instance of what Foucault (1980) would consider the extension of bio-power and the constitution of docile bodies through discourse.

Bodybuilding ethnopharmacologists and other gym members, though exhibiting some trust in knowledge systems as promulgated and disseminated by experts, generally argue that clinicians currently lack an 'adequate' knowledge of bodybuilding pharmaceuticals (Korkia and Stimson 1993: 123). Granted, many bodybuilders would welcome clinical assistance to arrive at a better understanding of drug effects and optimal drug usage. Bodybuilders are, so to speak, suitable 'targets' for the 'clinical gaze' (Foucault 1973). However, at present bodybuilding ethnopharmacologists are generally considered, by themselves and their peers, more knowledgeable than the typical doctor (Monaghan 1999b).

Knowledge of training and recuperation

For established (competent) bodybuilders, basic training principles are simply taken-for-granted through a process of social habituation. For instance, one experienced gym member claimed: 'bodybuilding isn't a rocket science, you lift heavier, you get bigger' (Field diary, 20 July 1995: Olympia Gym). However, becoming a bodybuilder – similar to processes of becoming within formal educational settings (cf. Salisbury 1994) – presupposes learning. Analytically, this embodiment of competence (especially when combined with force) has been linked to the construction of masculinity 'in schoolboy sport, in physical labour, in the cult fantasies of bodily perfection' (Connell 1983: 217, cited by Jefferson 1998: 80).

Within bodybuilding there are *general* rules concerning how and when to train; rules which must ultimately be tailored through personal experimentation. Correspondingly, while information is requisite for bodywork, self-transformation entails more than the conscious flow of information (Wacquant 1995a: 72). The following statement underscores the slow processual, investigative and complex nature of bodybuilding training:

> ... it takes a builder a long time to learn which ones [exercises] are best for him [*sic*], how best to mix and split them, when to increase or decrease weight and reps, and all the other thousand things he has to know to get the most from his workouts.
>
> (Gaines and Butler 1974: 72)

Bodybuilding argot lists a plethora of muscle-building exercises suitable for both men and women. Information concerning what these exercises are, reasons for executing them, alongside how and when to perform them, represents a body of knowledge which must be learnt by those striving for bodybuilding success.

Employing various training techniques presupposes knowledge of the body's anatomical structure. Bodybuilders participate in a full-body sport and they must know what muscles to train. Similar to non-Western ethnophysiological knowledge

(Manning and Fabrega 1973), the objectified body is conceived as fragmented and divisible. The body is divided into six basic parts or muscle groups; namely, chest (*'Pecs'*), arms, shoulders (*'Deltoids'* or *'Delts'*), abdominals (*'Abs'*), legs (*'Quads'*), and back (*'Lats'*). There are also subgroups within each of these major muscle groups and, correspondingly, many different exercises for these muscles.

Bodybuilders' ethnophysiological knowledge of the fragmented and divisible body is worth underscoring. As mentioned in the previous chapter, *'symmetry'* is an important judging criterion. All body-parts must be proportionately balanced, otherwise the bodybuilder may risk compromising bodily aesthetics. Being a *'toffee apple'* or *'bodybuilder on a stick'* (possessing a muscular torso that overshadows the legs), is an impediment to bodybuilding success.

Recuperation in bodybuilding, as in other strenuous sports, is deemed important because muscular hypertrophy only occurs *after* muscle-fibres have been broken down during vigorous isometric exercise. Experienced bodybuilders claim 'you don't grow in the gym'; hence, rest is sacrosanct. However, exercising different muscles on different days of the week (*'split routines'*) means that bodybuilders may lift weights practically every day without necessarily *'over-training'* (over-taxing the body's recuperative abilities and thus potential for muscle growth).

Various options are open to bodybuilders when planning the frequency of their training sessions. For instance, training *'two on, one off'* (two consecutive days followed by a day of rest) or adding an extra training day by doing *'three on, one off'* are popular options. More demanding regimens include *'double split, three on, one off'* (translation: two daily workouts for three days followed by one day of rest) (Wacquant 1995b: 164). Importantly, knowledge concerning the frequency of training must be tailored according to the particular strengths and weaknesses of each bodybuilder. This individualised knowledge may also figure in subcultural boundary maintenance:

Julie: You have to have a training programme for your three days on, two days off, two days on, one day off, make sure you rigorously train every body part. Some body parts may need training twice a week. You have to know your weaknesses and strengths, you got to know your body. You're learning about your body [...] you [might] need to work on your delts, they're weak, or your legs or hamstrings [...] The weight trainer [doesn't know all this], they just basically go to the gym and just do, just tone up, keep themselves in shape.

(Interview: Respondent 11)

In sum, ethnophysiological knowledge is requisite in successful bodybuilding. In ensuring ongoing muscular enhancement, bodybuilders must be aware of the various different muscle groups, exercises available, reasons for executing them, in addition to how and when to perform them. This detailed knowledge is instrumental in the construction of competent bodybuilding identity and building muscular bodies.

Ethnonutritional knowledge

Most illicit drug users attach little value to food, preferring instead to spend their money on drugs (Taylor 1993: 127). Bodybuilders, irrespective of their own drug user status, differ in this respect (Bolin 1992b). The centrality of diet, especially in contest preparation, means that 'ethnonutritional' knowledge (Mennell *et al.* 1992) is requisite. Bodybuilders' 'nutritional science' represents a rationalisation of conduct, the imposition of scientific norms and practices on everyday activities (Turner 1996: 22).

According to one of my respondents 'bodybuilding is ten years advanced on all other sports with nutrition, [other sports are] only copying what we've forgotten' (Interview: Respondent 13). Space constraints mean that this section merely skirts what is a vast area of bodybuilding. Nutritional supplementation is also noted, while acknowledging the limited role of these mass produced commodities relative to what many consider a more cost effective alternative; namely, steroids and analogous drugs.

Food: macro-nutrients and dietary techniques

Bodybuilders typically follow a high protein diet containing adequate complex carbohydrates and relatively little fat. The following exchange, which stresses the organic nature of the body, is also concordant with nutritional scientific thinking from the nineteenth century onwards where food is regarded as a form of fuel for the human body conceptualised as an engine (Turner 1996: 22):

LM: Why are you concerned about what you eat?

Mick: Because if I don't eat the right food, I don't grow, and if I don't grow I don't improve and if I don't improve I can't win competitions.

LM: So in what ways are you concerned?

Mick: With the extra food I eat I am concerned whether I got enough protein. The right amount of carbs [complex carbohydrates], not too much to get fat but enough to grow and keep my energy levels up so that I can train as hard as I can.

(Interview: Respondent 22)

Bodybuilders must be aware of the nutritional contents of specific foods and consume these foods. No doubt, this application of dietetic knowledge is illustrative of Foucault's concern with the rationalisation of behaviour, rendering bodybuilding an archetypal 'government of the body' (Turner 1991b). A non-competitor describes his meticulous dietary practices in the following terms:

Len: How I eat a meal now, when I go home I'll think 'right, I need 100 grams of carbohydrate', for example, '50 grams of protein'. And I'll have a cup of porridge, pint of skimmed milk. That takes me up to about 20 grams of protein and 100 grams of carbohydrate. Right, hang on, then I'll have half a dozen egg whites [yolks contain fat and are therefore discarded], or half a tin of tuna fish, and I think: 'that's given me just about 50 grams [of protein] and 100 grams of carbs'. No matter where I get them from, it could be two slices of bread, a smaller amount of porridge, tuna fish, chicken breast. It's all geared towards nutrition and not taste.

(Interview: Respondent 23)

Bodybuilders follow a plethora of dietary regimens and there is argument and controversy concerning the correct proportions of macro-nutrients in the diet (Bolin 1992b: 383). However, bodybuilders agree on the importance of dietary protein:

Len: [I'm concerned about what I eat] because it's 100 per cent of bodybuilding. Why bust your bollocks in the gym, excuse my French [sic], if you're not going to eat right? I mean, it's like your body cannot build muscle without protein. It doesn't matter, you can take a truck load of steroids a day, without that protein you can't do anything. You can't build a house without bricks can you? You just can't do anything. Totally ineffective. So, I think why bust my gut in the gym and spend my money on gear [steroids] if I'm not going to eat properly.

(Interview: Respondent 23)

One gram of protein per pound of body weight each day is touted as the general guideline in order to maintain a *positive nitrogen balance* (state of muscular growth). Further, because bodybuilders know the body cannot assimilate large amounts of protein in one meal (more than 50 grams per sitting is deemed excessive), protein intake must occur regularly. The bodybuilders' meals cannot be consumed in an anarchistic fashion; rather, they must be preplanned and scheduled in accord with ethnonutritional ideas on protein assimilation. A former competition bodybuilder of world championship standard commented:

> Sonny: I was making sure I was getting 25 to 30 grams of protein every two hours [...] my body weight was about two twenty [lbs] so I was aiming about 220 grams of protein a day. And knowing that you can only take in about 30 grams at one sitting, your body can only use in one go, I'd have, I'd have to split it up. So, I was having 25 to 30 grams every two hours, right throughout the day so I would be able to get in enough because I could have 150 grams in one meal but my body would only use 30 of it.
>
> (Interview: Respondent 17)

Before discussing nutritional supplementation, one final observation. Perhaps of most importance to bodybuilders during the last ten days of contest preparation are the practices known as *'carb-depleting'* and *'carb-loading'*. In manipulating their dietary intake of complex carbohydrates, competitors make the skin appear tight against their muscles thereby increasing their chances of success in a bodybuilding show. The rationale behind this technique is described below:

> Bill: The reason for depletion is that you try to fool the body into thinking you've just been through hard times – like a desert or something – and it thinks: 'Oh, right, we're getting these carbohydrates now' [during the re-loading stage]. So what happens is it [the body] stores the glycogen [digested carbohydrate] back in the muscles and it pushes the muscles right out due to the glycogen, stretches the skin, which has gone slowly down over three days [when depleting carbohydrates].
>
> (Interview: Respondent 24)

And, concerning the technicalities, timing and experimental nature of this dietary technique:

> Sonny: Carb-depleting which would be something like ten days out from the show, depleting the carbohydrates over a three day period. Then you have a day where you're taking in absolute zero, no carbohydrates at all, and then you start loading up slowly on carbohydrates [...]

> LM: So how many days would you [reload] for?

> Sonny: [...] Well, I'd say about five days, yeah somewhere about there, slowly each day [...] I'd increase it about 200 grams each day [...] what you got to do is make sure you got all your carbohydrates out of your body. So you have your workouts and once you finish your last workout for the show right, then you start carbing up. You have to try and deplete completely

[before you load up]. It's no good starting to carb up [otherwise]. You got to deplete completely then carb up and retain all the carbohydrates that you can right, ready for the show […]

LM: So it's a matter of timing, of getting your timing right?

Sonny: You got to get it spot on. And it's different for different people, they're different than me. I couldn't say to someone, 'look, do it that way', because it, it might be different for them. They might need an extra day or a day less or whatever, so you got to find out how long you're going to need to carb up for yourself.

(Interview: Respondent 17)

For bodybuilders, sophisticated ethnonutritional theorising represents a more or less 'correct' body of knowledge which must be modified through embodied social practice. Normative principles of *'carb-depleting'* and *'carb-loading'* cannot be specified in generalised terms but 'proof' that the tailored regimen works for the individual was offered by respondents in the form of observational data. Bill, who also shown me a photograph of himself competing in a bodybuilding competition, said: 'The skin over the muscles, it's like cling-film over a drum […] fills back out, the fibres all come bursting out. The skin is tight over your body' (Interview: Respondent 24).

The proof of the pudding may very well be in the eating. However, for individuals striving for bodybuilding success, food is geared towards nutrition and enhanced bodily aesthetics rather than taste. Consequently, for bodybuilders practising techniques such as *'carb-depleting'* and *'carb-loading'* the proof of the pudding is in the competing. Undoubtedly, modern competition bodybuilders look more muscular and defined than ever before (Klein 1992: 328). Employing sophisticated dietary techniques goes some way in accounting for this. Arguably, 'improvements' in bodybuilding, similar to the improvement in the health of the British population during the nineteenth and early twentieth centuries (McKeown 1979), owe more to dietary than medical developments.

Nutritional supplements

According to Turner (1996: 39), contemporary dietary management, and its relation to the external presentation of the body through, for example, scientific gymnastics and cosmetics, must be analysed in the context of changes in the production and distribution of commodities under a system of mass consumption. Here bodybuilders' ethnonutritional knowledge also extends to commercial supplements. Bodybuilding success, according to various respondents, and a plethora of globally distributed bodybuilding magazines, is dependent upon nutritional supplementation. According to one bodybuilder: 'you've got to take supplements if you want to get anywhere' (Interview: Respondent 9). Other interviewees asserted that the effective use of these products entails a detailed knowledge of the various substances available, their properties and effects. Consider, for example, the technical nature of Alan's supplement regimen:

Alan: I take Amino Acids – primarily to keep my nitrogen balance positive. Multi-vitamin mineral to make sure that I'm getting adequate sources. B Complex to aid the recuperation and keep my stress levels to a minimum. B6 and B12 to utilise and assimilate protein better and [...] Vitamin C – take an abundance of Vitamin C – 6 grams a day for the collagen effect – for the fact that they keep you [your skin] tight.

(Interview: Respondent 21)

Before describing the content of this knowledge, an important point should first be made. Namely, while many supplements are considered important adjuncts to the bodybuilding diet, widespread scepticism exists concerning the cost-effectiveness of these products compared to certain drugs. Fieldwork observations, recorded while training with bodybuilders who stressed the importance of supplementation during interviewing, indicate that drugs and 'basic' nutritional products are often considered more effective. Analysing such talk from within an accounts framework also suggests that steroid-using bodybuilders, similar to marihuana smokers who excuse their drug use on the grounds that it is cheaper than alcohol, may voice an appeal to defeasibility (Weinstein 1980: 580):

Bough: I was talking with Len who owns the Weider shop [sells bodybuilding paraphernalia]. He's been giving that 'Met-RX' [food supplement] a go. He said it's really good but it's expensive.

Mark: I think it works out at about £50 for a couple of weeks supply.

Bough: Yeah, you're supposed to have two sachets a day. At £2.50 a sachet – that's £5 a day, £35 a week.

Mark: It's a lot. You would be better getting some gear instead and a load of protein powder. That'd have more of an effect and it'd be a lot cheaper.

Bough: Yeah, at that price you might as well get a load of Deca [type of steroid].

(Field Diary, 16 December 1994: Temple Gym)

Similarly, Soccer maintained that profit-making entrepreneurs who mass produce these commodities are the primary beneficiaries. In using drug enhanced physiques to advertise and promote supplements, manufacturers reportedly profit at the expense of casual trainers who naively assume bodybuilding success is attainable by weight-training and using such products. Clearly, as suggested below, not all 'supplements' are deemed valuable. Bodybuilders' knowledge of supplementation may be considered scientific by those who possess it; however, being 'in the know' has more to do with knowing which products are valuable and those which are not:

Julie: It's quite scientific now. Very scientific, especially dieting and supplements. It's really hard to get to grips with, 'how much am I supposed to be taking here now? Oh, there's another new thing out on the market now'. But you got to know what to buy and what not to buy, because a lot of this is a waste of money [...] You know, it's gimmicks.

(Interview: Respondent 11)

Despite such gimmickry, it is evident that knowledge of supplements informs successful bodybuilding. Such knowledge, also linked to a 'care of the self' ethic (Foucault 1986) for many interviewees, is an additional element in the bodybuilders' commonsense world where participants consider themselves separate and distinct from irresponsible risk takers. These understandings are noted below, thereby completing an ethnographic overview of bodybuilders' ethnonutritional stock-of-knowledge:

'Nutritional supplementation' covers a whole spectrum of products ranging from protein and weight-gain drinks, to multivitamins and minerals. These products, legally obtained from a variety of sources including health-food shops, bodybuilding magazines, and pharmacies, are (as their name suggests) an adjunct to the diet. (Some supplements, which have a 'drug-like' effect, are viewed as 'training aids' and are therefore discussed in Chapter 6 on steroid accessory drugs.) Although by no means a substitute for the perceived 'healthy' diet endorsed and adhered to by many bodybuilders, ingesting these products on a regular and systematic basis is claimed to ensure an adequate supply of nutrients, resulting in maximum muscle growth:

Jack: Well, supplements, well they are what they are aren't they? Supplements. They're regarded as a supplement, not a main meal. So, what I do is use them to supplement my diet. That's all.

LM: And that helps your bodybuilding?

Jack: Oh yeah. It keeps the calories high, your blood sugar high, your amino acid pool high, your nitrogen retention. [They work] if you take them long enough. You've got to take them all the time. Like somebody will take a protein drink every couple of days, that's not going to do anything. Whatever you take like that, you got to take it a couple of times a day and consistently.

(Interview: Respondent 10)

Protein drinks are the most important supplement bodybuilders rely upon and are particularly useful for those unable to obtain sufficient amounts through food alone. By mixing this powdered supplement with milk, bodybuilders have a convenient and easily digestible source of protein, enabling them to ingest enough of this nutrient throughout the day. Indeed, because work obligations often interfere with the ability to eat regularly, supplements may be taken instead of meals, satisfying the bodybuilders' need to ingest nutrients at timed intervals:

Tim: I've got a good quality weight-gain protein drink, because as I say, I can't eat at regular times during the day and, when I work, well, I go four hours without a meal which is too long really. So I mean, if I can have a good quality protein and weight-gain drink half way through the first half of my shift.

(Interview: Respondent 16)

Although relatively expensive, many supplements such as vitamins and minerals are generally associated with a health-promoting effect both within the larger society and bodybuilding subculture. Annandale (1998: 18), following Beck (1992), notes how the manufacture of vitamins is an example of science turning towards the definition and management of the very risks which it itself produces. Vitamin C, for example, is described by bodybuilders as an antioxidant which neutralises toxins in the body caused by stress, environmental pollution and steroid use. Concerning the beneficial properties of Vitamin C, one drug-using bodybuilder said:

Gary: Yeah, it [keeps the colds away] more than anything, yeah. It's an anti-toxin as well. You know? Even if you didn't train your body builds up toxins anyway, but especially you know the stress involved during work or whatever, not just work, the training as well. And, the steroids actually build up toxins in your bloodstream as well like, yeah so Vitamin C helps to bind with it and pass it out through your system.

(Interview: Respondent 42)

In helping the body overcome possible steroid side effects, bodybuilders claim other supplements may be valuable:

Bill: I take calcium when I'm taking gear because the steroids, especially the oral steroids I think, they tend to take calcium and if you haven't got an adequate supply of calcium in the body, you will take it from the bones. And this is where you get osteoporosis and things.

(Interview: Respondent 24)

Bodybuilders experiencing significant strength gains claim Cod Liver Oil is a useful supplement for lubricating the knee and elbow joints. Evening Primrose Oil is also believed to confer numerous benefits for drug-using bodybuilders including its capacity to overcome insomnia and exert a therapeutic action on the liver.

Bodybuilders may make recourse to their supplementary regimen in order to buttress their view that they are responsible and health conscious. In this respect they are concerned with the principle that says one must 'take care of oneself' (Foucault 1986: 43); a principle which could serve the dual purpose of protecting the physical self (from possible harm through drugs, hard-training and stress) and the social self (imputations damaging to self-identity). For example one steroid injector, who reported turning to bodybuilding in order to overcome his heroin addiction, commented about the money he spent on supplements: 'After being a junkie and putting hundreds of pounds up your arm and doing harm to yourself, you don't really begrudge spending anything on something that's going to do you good, you know?' (Interview: Respondent 43).

Thus, as well as a convenient source of nutrition vital for fuelling and sustaining muscle growth, supplements are also believed to 'do you good'. Concerning their perceived biological benefits, certain supplements are claimed to protect against, or at least minimise, some of the potential health risks associated with steroids in particular and day-to-day living in general. Certainly, experienced bodybuilders claim the role of nutritional supplementation is frequently overemphasised in bodybuilding magazines. Nevertheless, there are products available which are considered a useful adjunct to the diet. Knowledge of supplementation, accorded scientific status by some participants, is therefore practically relevant. Furthermore, this knowledge, if acted upon, is ideologically significant. Even a reformed heroin addict, who became a bodybuilder and steroid injector, believed he was radically different from his previous self by referring to his current supplement programme.

Dedication

Fussell (1991) underscores the significance of dedication in successful body-building. He describes the response solicited from his two new gym mates, during the early stages of his bodybuilding career, after providing them with a drawing of the type of physique he aspired to create. He was informed ominously by his training partners that he needed to make the 'necessary adjustments'. This entailed altering his training routines, diet and supplementation programme. However, and above all, creating an accomplished bodybuilder's physique meant 'The Three D's [...] Dedication, Determination, Discipline. *That's* Bodybuilding' (Fussell 1991: 53).

Sacrifice and dedication, both in and out of the gym, render bodybuilding a radical lifestyle choice. One bodybuilder exclaimed: 'Bodybuilding ain't for a week or two then you get this [body], no it's for life! You've got to put your life into it' (Interview: Respondent 43). Other bodybuilders, concerned with subjugating and methodically developing their physiques, shared these sentiments: 'It is one of the hardest sports because it's not just a five minute thing. It's your life like, it's twenty four hours a day. To get into bodybuilding shape is literally twenty four hours a day, a real dedication' (Interview: Respondent 22).

Following the Foucauldian approach to bodily practices, Turner (1991b) states that disciplined regimens such as dietetic schedules represent a transposition of religious asceticism to secular space. As with boxers, this entails sacrifice and is

> tantamount to a form of secular bodily asceticism, that is, to paraphrase Max Weber's (1958: 172) well-known analysis in the *Protestant Ethic and the Spirit of Capitalism*, the methodical and rational subjection of individual impulse and desire to the pursuit of excellence through 'restless, continuous, systematic work' with and upon the body.
>
> (Wacquant 1995a: 76)

According to several respondents, most bodybuilders – by virtue of their dedication and commitment to the bodybuilding lifestyle – are comparable to religious converts. A gym owner commented: 'Like, when you consider our lifestyles, like we eat tidy [sensibly], or the majority do, eat tidy, train hard. Well, we literally live like monks' (Interview: Respondent 18). A female bodybuilder, committed to a draconian pre-contest diet exclaimed: 'bodybuilding is such a monastery!' Specific reference is made here to bodybuilders' dietary regulations. Dedication to personally imposed intense training, while important, is beyond the scope of this chapter.

Observing dietary regulations

Ethnonutritional knowledge must be acted upon to achieve bodybuilding success. For bodybuilders, the ability to follow dietary regulations (eating consistently throughout the day, ingesting food for its nutritional value rather than its palatability) entails dedication, making 'a real effort'. The following statement concerning a neophyte's improper diet highlights the significance of commitment (alongside knowledge):

> Bough [...] told me about Meredydd's diet: 'He said he'd made a real effort to eat before training. I asked him what he'd had that day and he said: "Cake". Fucking cake! Can you believe it! He's a fucking idiot. I asked him what sort of cake – maybe I'd got it wrong and he'd had a rice cake. No, it was a marzipan cake!'
>
> (Field Diary, 21 September 1994: Temple Gym)

Of course, active dieting is closely associated with women, with controlling the female body, thus possibly compromising male identity. As noted by Watson (2000: 80–7) this can be problematic for men not least because diet, along with exercise, requires an act of discipline possibly to the detriment of family and work obligations. However, in the context of other social obligations, the ability to sustain a commitment to diet (which, for bodybuilders, entails regular activity) may figure in the 'heroisation' of everyday life, which is simultaneously a process of 'masculinisation' (Featherstone 1992). During fieldwork Rod made the following positive remark about a junior competitor who later went on to win a national title and compete in the Mr. Universe (world championships):

> He's eating eight or nine times a day now. Like every hour and a half, and is making sure he gets about 50 grams of protein [per meal]. He's at college and he's got a friend who lives on the campus. He's got a food blender at his friend's place and a tub of protein. In between lectures they go back to have a protein drink.
>
> (Field Diary, 26 July 1994: Pumping Iron Gym)

Chapter 2 noted that diet is one criterion for identifying 'bodybuilders'. During interviewing Rod explained the difference between bodybuilders and weight trainers in terms of dedication to diet. As a gym owner Rod was identified to newcomers as a source of information on topics pertaining to productive bodybuilding. After providing neophytes with a basic information sheet describing the relevance of diet, he said:

Rod: So they'll come back to me and say: 'well, like, what do we do with all of this food then?' [...] And you say: 'well, right, you've got to eat six times a day'. And a few, it depends on how interested they are, you will encourage them to sort of take it up slowly and eventually get them dedicated, but the majority will just think: 'oh, bloody hell, I'm not eating that many times a day, I'll never have time!' And it's not that they haven't got time. Basically they can't be bothered.

(Interview: Respondent 18)

Willingness to not only eat regularly, but also consume unrefined, plain natural foods is also necessary for bodybuilding success. One bodybuilder said: 'I like a lot of junk food [...] but I know I have to eliminate junk food to look good' (Interview: Respondent 31). As part of the social construction of cultural identity, a parallel may be drawn here between bodybuilders' food selection and the Canadian Inuit's ethnonutritional preference for 'country' as opposed to 'store' food (Borre 1991). Just as Inuit identity can be expressed by hunting and eating seal meat to maintain physical and mental health (Borre 1991: 54), many bodybuilders construct their identity and achieve a sense of self-satisfaction through their determined efforts to eat 'correctly'.

In highlighting the religious significance of dietary regulations and food selection, several comparisons may also be drawn between Jewish and bodybuilding nutritional practices. Three obvious comparisons include: 1) the role of food regulations in defining group identity and social boundaries, 2) food selection and personal guilt and 3) internal group divisions/variability in adherence to diet:

Similar to semitic avoidance of pork, the elimination of certain types of food from the bodybuilding diet involves self-regulation, ecological factors and the retention of identity (*cf.* Grivetti and Pangborn 1974). High in grid and group (Douglas and Wildavsky 1982), dedicated bodybuilders are able to distinguish themselves from the general public (and other gym members) given their respective diets. Rod, for example, exclaimed: 'They [non-bodybuilders] don't realise that we just don't live their lifestyle. You know, ours is like baked potato, tuna or chicken and things like that, whereas theirs is a bloody good curry' (Interview: Respondent 18).

Second, self-imposed prohibitions against certain forbidden foods may cause guilt sufficient to deter consumption. Again, successful bodybuilding is comparable to Orthodox Judaism where *the thought* of eating pork may lead to a negative psychological state (Fieldhouse 1995: 128). A young female competition bodybuilder said: 'If I eat the wrong foods I can't cope with the guilt. The guilt sets in. Cracks me up. I get very guilty' (Interview: Respondent 11).

Third, while successful bodybuilding entails observing and abiding by dietary regulations, adherence largely depends upon the individual's formal competitive status. Bodybuilders preparing for a physique show are akin to Orthodox Jews who strictly follow standards of Kashruth (dietary regulations) based on biblical, rabbinical and customary rules (Fieldhouse 1995: 128). Those assuming the role of the non-competitor are similar to Reform Jews because they are often far more relaxed about their diets. These orientations are highly dynamic but also patterned. For example, following physique shows, bodybuilders, like boxers who 'pig out' after a fight, often withdraw their bodies temporarily from these regimens by eating pizza and confectionery (Wacquant 1995a: 80). Variable degrees of attachment to bodybuilding dietary practices may also reflect life course transitions (Bellaby 1990). A former competitor, who was approaching middle age, reflected upon his gradually shifting systems of relevances:

Bill: I read a wonderful quote today about a gourmet: 'Counting calories to a gourmet is like the hooker looking at her watch'. It's taking the pleasure of the act away really and so – that's it. As a bodybuilder you're never really happy with eating curries and things [...] you know it's wrong. As I get older I tend to do things more in moderation where I was absolute steel-willed before you know. And I'd say: 'nope, not eating that crap'.

(Interview: Respondent 24)

Dedication or obsessive addiction?

The athletic role has been thoroughly critiqued given its narrow definitions of success and failure and accompanying 'unhealthy' demands (Messner and Sabo 1994). Reflexive participants in bodybuilding, perhaps somewhat defensively, recognised the all consuming nature of their activities:

Mike: It does rule your day a bit [...] people say to me: 'you're a bit obsessive about it'. And I say: 'well, I'm not really obsessive. But you've got to make it a priority for your day, otherwise there's not much point doing it. If you're going to squeeze it in to some odd hour you've got here or there you're not going to get much out of it'. You know? You've got to give it ... the whole day has got to revolve around your training. Whether it's like your main thing or not, the fact is that you're not going to progress unless you're dedicated and give it priority.

(Interview: Respondent 15)

For observers the dedication evidenced by many bodybuilders in their everyday lives may seem excessive. 'To force your body to grow', writes Klein, 'necessitates [an] extreme preoccupation with diet, workout schedules, drugs, and so on' (1993: 260). The more 'extreme' commitment to bodybuilding, similar to highly marginal 'countercultural' female scarification, provokes repulsion by mainstream society and has been compared to self-harm practices like anorexia (Pitts 1998: 68). Making 'appeals to psychological drives' (Weinstein 1980: 580), clinicians are implicated in the authoritative construction of these negative images. Commitment to bodybuilding has recently been medicalised as a form of reverse anorexia termed 'muscle dysmorphia' (Pope *et al.* 1997).

As a 'monastery', the cult of muscularity undoubtedly demands disciplined self-regulation and adherence to ascetic bodily regimens. The 'hot/thick' commitment characteristic of traditional society is requisite in successful bodybuilding. Here parallels may also be drawn between bodybuilders and professional boxers (Wacquant 1995a: 78) who sometimes risk family life in their quest for success. Undoubtedly, relationships may be at risk but bodybuilders – similar to body modifiers interviewed by Sweetman (1999) – derive satisfaction, confidence and individuality from their absorbing body-centred activities. From one perspective, bodybuilding involves 'extreme preoccupation' and is obsessive in a pejorative sense but for many hard-core bodybuilders this attests to their own 'dedication' and is a source of self-identity.

Finally, it should be added that even the most disciplined of bodybuilders feel it is important periodically to pause from their ascetic lifestyle and enjoy other aspects of life. Sally, a high level competitor, quoted professional bodybuilder Mike Mentzer when she said: 'you should take time to smell the roses' (Interview: Respondent 19). Periods when members 'relax' and enjoy 'normal' activities (e.g. socialising in pubs with friends, drinking alcohol) is possible. More generally, this is a feature of commodity culture where individuals 'move between consumption and asceticism, between the "performance principle" and "letting go"' (Lupton 1997: 142). However, 'letting go' is severely limited among those prioritising success.

In summary, while individual bodybuilding goals may allow a more or less ascetic approach to training and dietary regimens, dedication is considered essential for those wishing to improve their bodies significantly. The biggest users of steroids and analogous drugs (physique competition bodybuilders) are also, by necessity, the most dedicated and self-disciplined members of the subculture. It follows that it is relatively unproblematic for these athletes to justify their steroid use. As stated by Rod: 'It [bodybuilding] is purely down to hard work, diet and dedication really. The more you put in, the more you get out. Bodybuilding and steroids in general really' (Interview: Respondent 18).

Finance

A key respondent mentioned the importance of finance specifically in relation to bodybuilding drugs. This facet of bodybuilding can prove expensive depending upon types of drugs used, frequency of use, duration, dosage and source. For example, research recently conducted among South Wales bodybuilders provides the approximate black market price of drug regimens administered by new and veteran steroid users, and a typical twelve week pre-contest protocol. These being £40, £140 and £370 respectively (Evans 1997: 56). However, as noted by a former competition bodybuilder, other costs are incurred:

Stan: It's a very expensive sport. 'Cause you're always feeding yourself and you become a big expense. I'm so expensive as a person because I have to keep myself in such a shape […] I used to spend £400 a month just on bodybuilding.

(Interview: Respondent 46)

The importance of finance in building a muscular body is, according to one respondent, often overlooked by non-participants. Instead, drugs are frequently considered the single most important ingredient:

Mark: As soon as you become a bodybuilder, people automatically think: 'well, he's on drugs' […] No-one actually says: 'oh well, oh, you've been there [at the gym] six days a week, you've spent all your money training, you've spent all your money on supplements, you watch your diet'. No-one ever says that anymore.

(Interview: Respondent 9)

Bodybuilding is similar to other modern sports: degree of involvement and the search for success brings proportionate costs. Training, diet, nutritional supplementation, drugs, clothes, a lifting-belt and straps are all costly. Contest preparation often proves very expensive. Alan told me he spent approximately £2,000 in preparation for the NABBA Mr. Britain bodybuilding championship; another competitor reportedly spent £10,000. Unless the athlete is black, competitors need to spend extra money on repeated applications of sun-tanning creams and sunbed sessions. This is necessary in order to prevent the body from looking 'washed out' under the powerful stage lighting. Competitors also need to purchase oils, posing briefs or bikini, razors and pay a subscription fee to a bodybuilding federation. The financial cost of bodybuilding (excluding money spent on 'extras' during pre-contest preparation) was noted by a high-level competitor:

John: They class it as a sport, as well as a hobby. The reason I don't class it as a hobby is because it's too expensive [...] To get anything out of bodybuilding you got to put in a lot of time, effort and a lot of expense. To use it as a hobby is too expensive [...] you got to eat enough to keep progressing, you got to eat, there's your supplements, you got to take vitamins, you got to take protein shakes whatever, and it's just too expensive to be used as a hobby. But to get the gains you got to be willing to pay that expense.

(Interview: Respondent 35)

Fortunately for John, he secured a sponsorship deal with a bodybuilding supplement manufacturer after winning an amateur world title. However, sponsorship is a luxury enjoyed by relatively few and even for those fortunate enough to obtain funding, this is only sufficient to contribute to the expense of contest preparation. Being a 'professional bodybuilder' in Wales or anywhere outside the United States means very little given bodybuilding's status as a 'Cinderella Sport' (i.e. its failure to be recognised as a sport within the larger society). A few bodybuilders mentioned the possible financial rewards of competition and national recognition as enjoyed by the sport's elite, but most considered such entrepreneurial activities beyond their own potential:

Jack: If I had a massive physique ... I'd utilise the physique and turn it to money. Dorian Yates [professional world I.F.B.B. champion], he could walk around just Great Britain doing seminars and earn a nice living, charge £400/500 a seminar. Do one a week and, you know, make a nice living out of it, see.

(Interview: Respondent 10)

The only competition bodybuilder interviewed for this study receiving financial reward (as opposed to receipt of expenses) for her sporting endeavours was Monique, a high standard Ms Figure-Fitness competitor. The body type which these bodybuilders strive to attain is more marketable than the Ms Physique category. Rather than creating an overtly muscular (androgynous) body, figure-fitness competitors cultivate an athletic look which is generally deemed more aesthetically pleasing in the eyes of both bodybuilding and non-bodybuilding men and women. Hence, international manufacturers of bodybuilding supplements, in using these competitors as models in their advertisements, are willing to provide financial backing and cash rewards for successful competitors.

Because most competitors receive no prize money, they undoubtedly incur the greatest costs. However, even for those non-competitors who are equally serious about their sport, bodybuilding can prove expensive. As commented by an interviewee who had only ever competed once during his lengthy bodybuilding career, this financial cost may be accompanied by a substantial opportunity cost:

Mike: If you added up the cost over the years you'd be frightened. Not in just what it cost you to eat and train and all the rest of it, but the more indirect things like opportunities you miss. Like you wouldn't take this job because there might not be a gym there, or you wouldn't want to work the overtime because I want to go training [...] I've missed out on loads of things [...] when I was in college and everyone was shooting off to 'Camp America', and I thought: 'bollocks to that. I'll be stuck in the middle of nowhere, not be able to train'. And all this sort of thing. You know? Little things like that. Yeah, it is expensive when you add it up over the number of years you actually train.

(Interview: Respondent 15)

The financial cost of bodybuilding was a recurrent theme during interviewing. Such expense may be affordable, however, given the nature of the dedicated bodybuilder's lifestyle. For example, committed bodybuilders tend to avoid alcohol. (Similarly, see Goldstein 1990: 90, who claims most of the bodybuilders sharing their experiences with him were very moderate drinkers or abstainers.) Rod, aware that alcohol in conjunction with steroids places an overload on the kidneys, stopped drinking altogether once he became a steroid user. Thus, although he was spending money on bodybuilding drugs, by eliminating his alcohol intake he reportedly made a net financial saving. This economy, coupled with the instrumental nature of bodybuilding, became a powerful rationale for this man when forced to justify his muscle-building to his wife. In response to his partner who felt that he was spending too much money on bodybuilding, Rod claimed to have said:

Rod: Well, how would you like it if, you know, I was a sort of average piss-artist, snooker player and sort of went to the pub like four or five times a week, you know, sort of spending like £70 a week pissing it up against the wall?

(Interview: Respondent 18)

Rejecting the working class conception of the pub oriented 'sporting man', Rod displayed the same somatic orientation as the privileged classes who treat the body as an aesthetic accomplishment and who 'engage in rites of an ascetic exaltation of sobriety and dietetic rigour' (Lupton 1997: 144). Making the body an ongoing project of the self is, however, dependent upon material security and advantage. While work may be an anathema to dedicated bodybuilders, because it interferes with serious training and regular nutritional intake, most bodybuilders and steroid users are employed (Lenehan *et al.* 1996, Williamson *et al.* 1993). The generality of this finding runs counter to the common perception of bodybuilders as unemployed men in search of a secure masculine identity. As one observer writes:

> ...as they [the bodybuilders] stressed to me, you could only afford bodybuilding's complicated regimes of diet and exercise if you had a reasonable wage coming in. Bodybuilders as gainfully employed, semi-bourgeois hobbyists? It doesn't exactly fit the grim post-industrial scenario.

> (Kane 1994: 2)

From a Foucauldian perspective this is indicative of the extent to which political investment in the body renders the body economically useful (Foucault 1979). Because most of my interviewees were in full-time employment, the necessary financial outlay for bodybuilding was more or less affordable. Some, however, supplemented their income with money earned as part-time doormen ('bouncers'). In this respect they acted as 'entrepreneurs in bodily capital' (Bourdieu 1986). Several interviewees normalised their expenditure by claiming bodybuilding was no more expensive than any other sport. Interestingly, one bodybuilder keen to present bodybuilding as a legitimate sport made recourse to this financial outlay, arguing that participants were bona fide athletes.

In summary, finance is an important parameter for successful bodybuilding. Of course, similar to knowledge and dedication, the cost of bodybuilding is proportionate to the individual's desire for success. For those religiously embracing the bodybuilding lifestyle, finance is a salient consideration. Monetary outlay, and the opportunity cost of bodybuilding, may be substantial. Bodybuilding, for the vast majority of competitors, incurs a large financial outlay with no monetary return such as prize money or sponsorship. The ability to afford expensive leisure activities, as noted by McDonald-Walker (1998) in her study of British Bikers, may bolster 'respectable' identities in the face of negative stereotyping.

Genetics

While biology does not determine the social, creative embodied social practice occurs within variable biological limits. As Shilling (1993: 10–11) says: 'Human bodies are taken up and transformed as a result of living in society, but they remain material, physical and biological entities'. Bodybuilders' understandings are congruent with this theorisation. For example, Mr. Universe Mike Mentzer has often made the point that 'choosing the right parents' is the surest way to bodybuilding success, all the rest is just following through on what nature has bestowed upon the athlete (Kennedy 1983: 7). According to bodybuilders, '*genetics*' determine the number and distribution of muscle cells in the material body and thus the possibility of achieving bodybuilding success. A former professional bodybuilding judge explained the general relevance of this gender-wide parameter:

Pete: See, it doesn't matter who you are, what you are, what height you are, etc., etc., if Mother Nature hasn't put the muscle cells there, there's nothing else going to make the muscle grow is it? So if you're blessed with the right genetics, if you pick the right parents and you're prepared to work then you're way ahead of everyone else.

(Interview: Respondent 13)

Soccer claimed his '*genetics*' were an impediment to obtaining the type of physique he aspired to create. Physique-enhancing drugs were deemed necessary in order to compensate for what he considered a poor genetic inheritance. The following quote, which is illustrative, is noteworthy for another reason. Experienced bodybuilders maintain that gauging one's own genetics requires time and patience. Incidentally, this is one of the main reasons why many bodybuilders claim neophytes should postpone drug-taking for as long as possible. Otherwise, they will never know how good they can become without drugs:

Soccer: My reason for training was to obtain what I considered to be the perfect physique [...] And I was under the illusion that I would achieve this physique somewhere around the two year mark and I have since found that because, maybe of my genetics, that for me personally that I would never achieve that physique without taking assistance by drugs.

(Interview: Respondent 7)

Although practically all first-class competition bodybuilders use or have used steroids (Gaines and Butler 1974: 73), according to today's demanding standards the type of 'look' necessary to win a championship *also* requires the athlete to be 'genetically blessed': 'You've got to have the genetics [to be a top bodybuilder] and be there [physically], or half way there before you pick a weight up' (Interview: Respondent 10).

Bodybuilders accept that if an individual is genetically gifted, they will be able to develop a reasonably good competition standard physique without drugs provided they observe other parameters for successful bodybuilding. Given the prevalence of drugs, however, it is widely felt that a genetically gifted drug-free bodybuilder is unlikely to secure a prestigious title. According to bodybuilders the current standard of physique means that somebody would have to be 'the most genetically gifted person on the planet' to build a championship physique without some form of 'assistance'. Even then, a drug enhanced bodybuilder with inferior '*genetics*' may very well win:

Mike: I've been training for something like seventeen coming up for eighteen years and I've not really known anyone that's built a proper sort of competition physique without some form of assistance (laughs) shall we say.

LM: So you don't think it is possible to build that sort of physique naturally [without drugs]?

Mike: Not unless you're the most genetically gifted person on this planet, and even then the second most gifted person on the planet will beat you if he uses steroids.

(Interview: Respondent 15)

With the 'correct' use of chemicals a '*genetic freak*' simply becomes '*awesome*' (developed beyond belief) provided they are also knowledgeable, dedicated and solvent. Bodybuilders maintain that certain drugs only enhance the effectiveness of hard training and diet among those with a natural affinity for accruing muscle. Accordingly, while 'professional bodybuilding [is] a sport nearly synonymous with steroid use' (Todd 1987: 101), many participants assert that if drugs were removed from their sport tomorrow, there would be no change in the world rankings. The sport's elite, though not as muscular as they are today, would still be the best.

Drugs are, of course, part of the bodybuilding scene. However, in underscoring the perceived significance of '*genetics*', consider the following talk:

Soccer: There's this one bloke who claims he is natural – a big bastard he is – and I have it on good authority from several reliable people I know that he's never touched the gear [steroids]. He's just a genetic freak. His body responds to the training very well. This bloke entered the Mr. Wales. It wasn't NABBA [...] the standard wasn't as good as NABBA, but the competitors were still good though. Anyway, six weeks prior to entering he decided to start training legs and he was still good enough to win. On stage it was a flip of a coin whether it'd be him or this other bloke – it was that close. As it happened he won, but the bloke who came second said that he spent £500 prior to the show on gear.

(Field Diary, 20 March 1995: Olympia Gym)

And:

It was Len's birthday, and so to celebrate the occasion we went for a meal. While sitting next to Len I asked him about his friend, Sam. From the conversation it emerged that Sam ignored all the necessary precepts for bodybuilding and yet he had an impressive physique. The following exchange occurred:

LM: Sam drinks loads of beer, hardly eats at the weekend and yet looks like that [very muscular]. What [drugs] is he taking then?

Len: He's just got genetics coming out of his ear-holes. You know the old owner of Thor's Gym? Three weeks after Sam started training the gym owner asked him if he'd be going in for a show soon. He's just a naturally muscular guy. Only has to look at a weight and he grows. He eats shit – everything is fried. Even fried Chinese food. To him bodybuilding is just a hobby, he hasn't got that commitment but seeing as he doesn't compete he doesn't need to be so dedicated and yet still look fantastic. Although normally he eats shit he's been having some decent tidy grub like pasta, baked potatoes and chicken breasts over the last few days as he's been staying over at mine [Len's home]. After one day you could see the difference in his physique – fuller, with veins popping out of his chest. He's just a natural. Genetic freak. In the gym he can do just three sets of curls for biceps and think: 'Aggh, fuck it'. Walk away from it and grow just from doing that!

(Field Diary, 20 May 1995: Restaurant)

Finally, bodybuilders maintain that drug effectiveness is mediated by '*genetics*' (see Chapter 5). For example, I told Alan I had talked with several people who had experimented unsuccessfully with Human Growth Hormone. Alan explained: 'I think it depends on who you are, how your body is genetically gifted' (Interview: Respondent 21). Ethnopharmacologists claim drug side effects also vary according to individual '*genetics*'. According to their theorising, using drugs to compensate for genetic shortcomings may result in a disproportionately high risk-to-benefit ratio, possibly leading to steroid abuse.

In sum, according to bodybuilders' subcultural systems of relevances, dedication, knowledge and finance are necessary but not sufficient in developing a championship standard body. Drugs are also of limited value given the importance of '*genetics*'. Bodybuilders maintain that natural bodily potential, for both men and women, has a significant bearing upon success (Lowe 1998: 22). Even so, while the body may have inherent genetic limitations, 'nature' is not determinant and the hierarchy of bodybuilding, unlike caste and aristocracy, cannot simply be attributed to (biological) inheritance (Bellaby 1990: 470). Dedicated bodybuilders, as enterprising and technically innovative individualists, push back 'natural' bodily limits and displace subcultural divisions based upon physical appearance. Moreover, impermanent and fluid social differences, although often allocated to a select few women in the bureaucracy of elite competition bodybuilding (Lowe 1998: 54), suggest the culture of bodybuilders is not unambiguously hierarchical. Correspondingly, and as will emerge in the next chapter, bodybuilders' shifting orientations to types of muscular body and ultimately self-other imposed risks may be more variegated and dynamic than intimated by the culture of risk approach and critical feminist studies.

Conclusion

Bodybuilders' subcultural systems of relevances and typifications, which incorporate but which also extend beyond drug-taking, provide materials which are instrumental in the social construction of 'appropriate' bodies and identities. Parameters for 'successful' bodybuilding – knowledge, dedication, finance and genetics – constitute bodybuilders' commonsense understandings of reality. Here, individuals as bodybuilders are 'at home' (Schutz 1964: 252). In their common subcultural surroundings, bodybuilders are able to take their everyday (deviant/ risky) activities for granted (Berger and Luckmann 1966, Schutz 1967) and eschew stigmatising labels. Embodying powerful ideologies of asceticism, self-discipline and control, committed bodybuilders are able to construct a moral image 'in a culture which is intent upon self-promotion and achieving "the look"' (Lupton 1997: 146).

In proposing a four part typology for successful bodybuilding, the common typifications and relevances in terms of which *bodybuilders define their situation* were detailed. As stated by Schutz: 'such a general framework is experienced by the individual members in terms of institutionalizations to be interiorized, and the individual has to define his [*sic*] personal unique situation by using the institutionalised pattern for the realisation of his particular personal interests' (1964: 253). However, what are these particular personal interests through which individuals qua bodybuilders define their personal unique situation? Questioning the claim that bodybuilding, drug-taking and risk can be theorised adequately in terms of antecedent personal and gender insecurity (Klein 1995), the next chapter goes some way towards answering this question by documenting the spatially and temporally contingent task of creating 'the perfect body'.

Chapter 4

Creating 'the perfect body': a variable project

In conceptualising risk in the health field, there is a tendency to label social behaviour according to stereotyped constructs of personal inadequacy (Williams *et al.* 1995: 120). Negative labelling is intimately related to the construction of 'stigma theory': an ideology formulated to explain the inferiority of the discredited and the danger they represent (Goffman 1968: 15). Studies homogenising the variable project of bodybuilding are examples of stigma theory. Adopting a psycho-analytic stance, Klein states that 'bodybuilding is, at the very least, a subculture whose [male and female] practitioners suffer from large doses of insecurity; hence, compensation through self-presentation of power to the outside world' (1993: 174). Allegedly caused by antecedent personal and/or gender inadequacy and a masculinity-in-crisis within the larger society, bodybuilding and drug-taking represent an 'atavistic' strategy for concealing self-perceived flaws. In particular, the erosion of men's traditional occupationally derived privileges in a post-industrial order prompts some to compensate for their feelings of powerlessness by embodying the physical trappings of 'hegemonic masculinity'. Accordingly, 'the muscular body' becomes synonymous with the culturally idealised masculine/ powerful/self-assured body (Klein 1993: 242).

'There are in principle always an indefinite number of theories that fit the facts more or less adequately' (Hesse 1980: viii). Correspondingly, muscle-building (and attendant 'risky' practices such as steroid abuse) may be linked not only to gender anxieties within ornamental culture (Faludi 1999), but also to ontological and class insecurity (Wacquant 1995b), the constitution of 'docile' bodies through discourse (Foucault 1980), and a culture of narcissism (Lasch 1980). Because many bodybuilders inject steroids, bodybuilding could, in following Douglas and

Calvez (1990), also be theorised in terms of cultural isolation or fatalism. More positively, the unitary act of bodybuilding, may be theorised in terms of the reflexivity of self and a proliferation of 'body regimes' in late modernity (Giddens 1991), or the representational significance of the (homogenised) exercised and dieted fe/male body within postmodernity (Glassner 1990), consumer culture (Featherstone 1991), or somatic culture (Wachter 1984). And, in following Shilling's (1993) extension of Bourdieu's analysis of cultural and embodied capital to the sociology of the body, there is the manner in which sport renders the unfinished object of the human body a social project and bearer of symbolic value (Shilling 1993: 128).

While existing sociological theory is noteworthy, and may be invoked to explain bodybuilding at various different levels of abstraction, it rarely takes as its starting point the embodied experiences of individuals within their own social worlds (Watson *et al.* 1995). In theorising bodybuilding, drugs and risk, this chapter takes as its starting point male participants' shared 'in-order-to motive' (Schutz 1967). (As will become apparent, men are purposively selected as a 'critical case' rendering my argument feasible when accounting for women's participation in bodybuilding.) While many different, overlapping and often contradictory reasons *may* be invoked for the (sub)cultural phenomenon of bodybuilding and individual predilections for accruing muscle, what is certain is that all bodybuilders are united in the ongoing project of enhancing bodily aesthetics. In short, bodybuilding is undertaken by embodied social agents – within a carnal version of what Bourdieu (1992) would term the '*habitus*' (Crossley 1995: 56) – 'in-order-to' create 'the perfect body'.

If the body is the point at which all muscle enthusiasts converge, then this is also their point of departure. Building a lean muscular body is a project which unifies bodybuilders, but also a source of contrast given many different visions of physical perfection. In this highly individualised domain, 'bodybuilder' (a less than satisfactory referent according to some members) is a heterogeneous category. Participants may even pursue their own muscle agenda independent of the dynamic and frequently contested 'objective' criteria dictated by their various different competition federations (Guthrie and Castelnuovo 1992: 406). Conceptions of 'physical perfection' are spatially and temporally contingent, varying from one individual to the next and also for the same individual during the course of their bodybuilding career.

For 'hard-core' bodybuilders (Mansfield and McGinn 1993), conceptions of 'the perfect body' are dependent upon a subculturally informed 'ethnophysiological' (Manning and Fabrega 1973: 257) appreciation of 'excessive' muscularity. Grounded in data (Glaser and Strauss 1967), the following 'grapples with theoretical issues' (Frank 1995: 187) by questioning the critical feminist claim that bodybuilding is a 'knee-jerk' response to psychosocial forces and a wish to embody hegemonic masculinity. Stigmatised rather than idealised by the mainstream public, drug assisted 1990s physique bodybuilding (at least at regional and national level competitions and beyond) is analogous with various non-Western ethnophysiological practices e.g. neck-stretching, cranial deformation, ornamentation of the earlobes and insertion of lip discs (*cf.* Brain 1979, Polhemous 1978). Shaping members' socially acquired 'ways of looking', bodybuilding ethnophysiology also enables subcultural aesthetes to differentiate and evaluate different bodies, parts of bodies, as well as providing a knowledge of what is required to achieve a certain body type. Correspondingly, bodybuilders' learnt ways of looking *at* bodies informs *their* decision to approximate the look of a particular soma type and thus *their willingness* to commit themselves to bodybuilding over time.

Becoming and remaining a bodybuilder, it will be argued, is only possible if the individual has arrived at a conception of the meaning of the activity and perceptions and judgements of types of muscular body which make ongoing physical development possible and desirable (similarly, see Becker 1963). In discussing the importance of acquired ethnophysiology in the *transmogrification* of the physical body, a direct critique is levelled against feminist analyses (Gillett and White 1992, Klein 1993, White and Gillett 1994) and other critical work on this topic (e.g. Day 1990). In short, it highlights the limitations and blind spots of existing approaches which treat 'bodybuilder' as a singular category, and which explain bodybuilding, drugs and risk in terms of the dual interplay of the masculinist imagery of 'the muscular body' and antecedent sociocultural forces perceived to be beyond individual control (Gillett and White 1992: 366).

Viewed through the lens of social phenomenology, motives and dispositions (not *pre*-dispositions) for (chemical) bodybuilding emerge during the course of the individual's experience. Ongoing practical involvement in the bodybuilding habitus in time produces motivations for accruing 'excessive' muscularity (the *sine qua non* of the dedicated bodybuilder) rather than the other way round. Vague impulses and desires – in this case, most frequently a wish to 'tone up' and look athletic, fit, young and sexually attractive (*cf.* Monaghan *et al.* 1998) – are transformed into definite patterns of action through the subcultural interpretation or 'artistic deciphering' (Bourdieu *et al.* 1991) of what non-participants consider a homogenous entity. This argument, which recognises the body is social and the social is embodied (Crossley 1995), is advanced by pluralising 'the muscular body' and highlighting the importance of social process.

Pluralising 'the muscular body' or 'ways of looking'

In critically engaging a particular strand of feminist literature, a caveat is required. Documenting bodybuilding ethnophysiology and members' heterogeneous body-projects does not, by itself, place a question mark against existing knowledge claims. The following could merely be taken to suggest that academics should be more sensitive to differences in the bodybuilding community. However, if the types of muscular bodies to which 1990s bodybuilders (not weight trainers) orient themselves are not culturally prescribed but are instead stigmatised, then bodybuilding cannot be theorised adequately in terms of an *antecedent* culturally endorsed image i.e. 'the muscular (masculine) body'. Of course, a general masculine will to be muscular *may* figure in the genesis and sustainability of bodywork, but then again it may not (Glassner 1990). In accounting for the ongoing variable project of bodybuilding, I feel a more satisfactory account – which is attentive to the diversity of members' meanings – must recognise that in the sport and art of bodybuilding, 'aesthetic pleasure presupposes learning and, in any particular case, learning by habit and *exercise*' (Bourdieu *et al.* 1991: 109, emphasis added).

In contrast to other types of weight trainer, bodybuilders typically pluralise 'the muscular body'. The individual bodybuilder's desire to emulate or approximate the 'look' *of* a particular soma type is therefore intimately tied to the lived body's socially acquired 'ways of looking' *at* physical bodies. This statement, which differentiates between the body as *Korper* and *Leib* (Turner 1992), is concordant with Merleau-Ponty's (1962) phenomenology of embodiment. According to Merleau-Ponty the body-subject's primary relation to the environment consists in practical competence. In short, there is a primacy of practical over theoretical or abstract ways of being in the world (Crossley 1995: 53). Within bodybuilding subculture, members' practical purposes at hand render 'the muscular body' (*Korper*) a variegated and thus heterogeneous entity rather than an undifferentiated object which supposedly signifies hegemonic masculinity to the outside world. Academic writings on bodybuilding, offering a reading of the singular 'muscular body' at the level of cultural signification, therefore ride roughshod over complex social reality.

Consider the following extract. Various issues and themes emerge, including Soccer's and Alan's shared ability to differentiate and evaluate *different types of* muscular body. These 'ethnophysiological' understandings enable bodybuilders to discern between various types of body which are, for all practical purposes, homogeneous to non-initiates but more or less aesthetically pleasing from their acquired viewpoints:

Soccer was talking about some of the physiques displayed on posters in the gym reception. There was a picture of Dorian Yates [current professional world champion].

Soccer: My friend saw him at a seminar. I think he was about 23stone [...] I suppose it's a bit difficult to gauge how big he is from that picture since there's nothing there to put it into scale. I suppose you'd get a good idea if you put Linford Christie there. I mean, Christie isn't a small man. If he was stood next to that [Dorian] though, he'd be dwarfed ... I wouldn't want to look like that [Dorian]. Then again, I would for a year so I could earn loads of money, get the prestige, give seminars, but I wouldn't be happy with the way I looked. I'd slim down to that after a year [pointing to a picture of a less well known professional bodybuilder who was not as muscular as Dorian Yates, but who was still extremely muscular by anybody's standards]. More of a natural physique as opposed to that [Dorian]. Obviously that [smaller bodybuilder] isn't natural [i.e. he uses steroids] but it's more pleasing to the eye in my opinion [...]

Alan, the gym owner and competitor of world amateur standard, walked in.

Soccer: I was just talking to Lee, saying how I'd prefer to look like that [smaller bodybuilder] than that [Dorian]. At least with this physique [smaller bodybuilder] you could still wear clothes and not look fucking ridiculous [in your day to day interactions with the public]. I'd like to be more like him there, Bob Paris. He's very symmetrical, not a lump like Dorian Yates [...] Paris has got a good physique, not massive [by today's competition standards] but very symmetrical.

Alan: Yeah, in the Mr. Olympia in the 80s when he competed it was said he was gonna be the new face of bodybuilding [Alan went on to talk about the issue of size in bodybuilding]. No doubt, Dorian Yates is the best there is, but for me bodybuilding is not about getting as big as you can get. I'm not a big guy anyway. Then again, because of my height [he's 5′6″] I'd look like a wardrobe if I was carrying a load of mass. I create the illusion that I'm big on stage though. Bodybuilding is all about illusion. Sculpting your body, carving out a shape which looks impressive but which, in reality, isn't that big.

(Field Diary, 24 February 1995: Al's Gym)

As well as rejecting the idea that sheer size is the primary goal of bodybuilding (*cf.* Klein 1993: 246), the national physique champion quoted below also pluralised 'the muscular body'. And, given sensitivity to the objective attitudes of generalised others (Mead 1934), viz. the mainstream public's disparagement, this narrator attempted to reconcile competing definitions of 'the body beautiful':

Rod: I've never actually seen Dorian Yates in the flesh but I think, to be honest, I don't think [name of bodybuilding entrepreneurs] are realising the image they're putting on bodybuilding and the way that they're starting to frighten the public off. If they had somebody like sort of Flex Wheeler who has a nice shape and had him as a winner [of the Mr. Olympia]. He had nice genetics [natural predisposition to accruing muscle] before he started, you know, and a lovely shape. You know, like Shawn Ray as well. He enters [competitions] at about 14 stone. And then you've got Dorian Yates who enters at like 20 stone and he walks on stage and scares the shit out of everybody! [...] I think a classic physique is like Francis Benfatto, the French one. There's superb quality. He'll enter at about 13 stone and he had beautiful genetics and yet he wouldn't get a look in [rank highly in the competitions]. It's got to be like this mass of muscle, flesh and veins, you know, nothing beautiful about it like. It's just basically like a big fuck-off body like! And [name of bodybuilding entrepreneurs] who've brought bodybuilding into the public eye over the last say, forty years, have turned round and spoilt it all by doing this now. Like with Arnold Schwarzenegger, everybody accepted that he was sort of big, but [...] Dorian Yates [is massive]. You get Dorian Yates and you're talking holy shit! It's like seeing two lots of Shawn Ray!

(Interview: Respondent 18)

Sam Fussell's bodybuilding narrative (1991: 102–4) similarly highlights the heterogeneity of bodybuilders' body-projects ('muscular bodies') and variable subcultural perceptions. Not only does the protagonist refer to different types of muscular body, this member's specific value-orientation means that from his perspective 'mass' (sheer size) is prioritised over 'class' (typically smaller, more 'elegant' and defined musculature). At a time when the championship standard male physique veered towards the chiselled or cut look, this man was not happy:

'... Now, you look at these shrunken poodles that pass for Mr. Universe these days', he [Macon] said, showing me a well-thumbed magazine with a particularly emaciated specimen in green posing trunks on its cover [...] 'I'll tell you somethin': You just give me one of them starvin' Biafrans, and I'll show you muscle striations. I mean have you seen the abs and intercostals on some of them guys? [...]' Macon continued. 'It's just like I told you yesterday son, these things go in cycles. All you got to do is open a book and examine history. Now, son, the late sixties and early seventies were a time when size ruled, with them Arnold and Serge Olivas and Lou Ferrignos. Then – kind of like what the good book says – a darkness fell over the land, 'cause the mid-seventies came and those Frank Zanes and sunken-cheeked foreigners ruled the stage. I mean, why would anybody in their right mind pay to see some guy with a Chippendale's physique? But now, thanks to Lee Haney, we might be coming back to good times, Arnold times, ...'

For the iron cognoscenti, particular bodies displayed by specific individuals (e.g. Frank Zane, Lee Haney), or more generalised figures of popular culture (e.g. 'the Chippendales'), are of one ethnophysiological type or another. Such categorisation or typification entails (among other things) an acquired knowledge of the properties of body parts and somatic features. In focusing upon various physical charact-eristics, participants employ ethnophysiological concepts as described in the previous chapter. Foucault's analysis of the 'disciplining' of bodies, and the signi-ficance of technologies of power in the institutional elaboration of gendered bodily practices, could be considered particularly relevant in this sporting context. However, the important (compatible and complementary) point being stressed here is that these indigenous terms – employed by the 'pictorially competent' (Bourdieu *et al.* 1991) when looking *at* muscular bodies – are meaningful to members but foreign to out-groups (Aoki 1996: 60).

In distinguishing between different bodies and parts of bodies, participants describe the features of various physiques displayed at bodybuilding competitions, in the gyms, magazines, etc. During interactions with significant others, neophytes also arrive at an acquired appreciation of types of muscular body in terms of their overall visual impact. In short, through a process of identification they learn to define different types of muscular body exhibited by contemporaries and predecessors as more or less aesthetically pleasing. As might be anticipated from Crossley's (1995) extension of Bourdieu's (1992) concept of the *habitus* to a 'carnal sociology of the body', types of muscular body *may* then be consciously set as projects for the self. The bodybuilding *habitus* effectively becomes 'the basis of choice [and] a structure of preferences' (Crossley 1995: 56).

These choices are made within limits of practicability (Schutz 1967: 73) and are intimately associated with risk (Fox 1998: 679). Experienced bodybuilders claim vigorous exercise and proper nutrition help create certain types of bodybuilding physique only if accompanied by drug-taking. This has implications when assessing the utility of the culture of risk approach (*cf.* Bloor 1995: 94). From an embodied perspective, self-imposed risks cannot simply be theorised in terms of adherence to group norms (as outlined in Chapter 2). Rather, shifting perspectives about types of muscular body and the means of attaining such bodies underpin risk practices (similarly, see Watson, 2000, on male embodiment and health practices).

As described in Chapter 3, '*genetics*' also delineate limits of practicability. If every (biological) body is different, the look an individual bodybuilder can achieve will always be an approximation of any idealised image selected from a plethora of body types:

Gary: You look at bodybuilders in magazines and I think I wouldn't mind having a body like that, but then every body type is different so it's really hard to picture yourself what you're going to look like. I suppose everyone does sort of picture what they'd like to look like, but what you'd like to look like and what you do look like is completely different.

(Interview: Respondent 42)

Doug: I want to look like this, you know, him. Or, yeah, I want to be like that. But you've no idea how it's going to turn out. It never turns out the way you think it's going to turn out. Unless you're progressing through body-building, you don't tend to realise this. Each bodybuilder is an individual.

(Interview: Respondent 29)

Clearly, each bodybuilder is an individual. Contrary to the common assumption in subcultural analyses, participation does not entail a transitory loss of self or individuality (*cf.* Widdicombe and Wooffitt 1995: 139). Rather, and as will emerge in the next chapter on managing steroid risks, 'individuality' is emphasised. Of course, the heterogeneity implied by this individuality does not obviate shared meaning; it is possible to clarify what is meant by 'the muscular body' among bodybuilders. Here reference should be made to Table 4.1. This typology of different male muscular bodies includes the names of specific figures or individuals exemplifying particular soma types (including types of muscular bodies which differ from bodybuilding physiques and against which bodybuilders contrast and thus define themselves). The typology not only highlights the limitations of critical feminist work on bodybuilding, but also other academic readings where it is claimed bodybuilding emphasises one ideal body type and exhibits a trend towards uniformity and sameness (Day 1990: 50–1).

Cultural analysts, who typically view the body as a target and object, or 'effect', of discourse would perhaps consider these category differences irrelevant. While significant for participants, cannot the whole panoply of types have the same, or similar social psychological underpinnings (just as, say, bulimia and anorexia may have similar psychosocial determinants)? Certainly, bodywork could be

Table 4.1 A typology of male muscular bodies

Competition Standard Bodybuilding Physiques (Sizeably Muscular and Exceptionally Lean):

Ripped, Awesome Mass Monster (e.g. Dorian Yates)
Ripped, Extremely Vascular Mass Monster (e.g. Paul Dillett)
Ripped, Massive and Classy (e.g. Kevin Levrone)
Ultra Ripped/Cut/Striated and Big (e.g. Andreas Muntzer)
Class with Perfect Symmetry (e.g. Bob Paris, Shawn Ray, Flex Wheeler)
Class from the Past (e.g. Frank Zane)
Mass from the Past (e.g. Arnold Schwarzenegger)

Powerful Looking Bodies (Sizeably Muscular but Lacking Definition)

Smooth Looking Physique Competitors in the Off-Season
Strength Athletes, e.g. Power-Lifters, Olympic Weight-Lifters, World Strongest
    Man Competitors
Wrestlers or Rugby Players

Athletically Muscular/Toned Bodies (Moderately Muscular and Typically Fairly Lean):

Natural or Non-Drug Enhanced Competition Bodybuilders
Champion Bodybuilders in the 1950s
Neophyte Bodybuilders
Fitness Oriented Weight Trainers
The Sprinter (e.g. Linford Christie) or the Chippendale
The Long Distance Runner or the Swimmer
Olympic Gymnast
Naturally Lean Men

---

considered the 'psychopathological' crystallisation of culture, where bodies are constrained and trained in docility and obedience (Bordo 1993). However, such theorising must presuppose some notion of a body-subject and communicative intersubjectivity which is facilitated through symbolic processes (Crossley 1996: 110). Phenomenologically speaking, the body is not simply an object in the social world but 'a sentient being whose primary relation to its environment should be understood in terms of this meaningful sentience' (Crossley 1995: 47). If the body's being-in-the-world is mediated through perceptual meaning, and meanings are subject to re-definitions, re-locations and re-alignments (Blumer 1969), social theorists should concern themselves with the concrete practices through which real bodies are produced. Bodybuilders, it would seem, are not 'cultural dopes' (Garfinkel 1967) whose actions are 'caused' in a mechanical way by an external force (though they could, in 'bad faith' [Sartre 1958], view themselves and others as determined objects through a retrospective glance). Rather, they are embodied social agents who are communicative and practical beings, drawing upon a common habitus (Shilling 1993: 129) which is amenable to sociological study (Crossley 1995: 60–1).

Contrary to theories explaining bodybuilding in terms of the masculinist imagery of 'the muscular body' and psychosocial forces perceived to be beyond individual control, the following considers the importance of social process and acquired ethnophysiology in the creation and recreation of 'Sizeably Muscular and Exceptionally Lean Bodybuilding Physiques'.

The importance of social process

Various contributors assert the agency of bodies in social processes (Connell 1995, Gatens 1996), arguing for a theoretical position in which bodies are seen as sharing in social agency, in generating and shaping courses of conduct (Watson 1998: 177). My ethnographic observations strongly suggest that bodybuilders' ways of looking at bodies – rendering ongoing muscular enhancement and regularised instrumental drug use possible and desirable – are acquired over time in the bodybuilding habitus. Social process, changing embodied perceptions and sub-cultural affiliation are therefore important. In claiming bodybuilders qua social agents possess a subculturally learnt system of cognitive and motivating structures (Shilling 1993), the following notes the extent to which their 'indigenous' perceptions contrast with non-members' (and marginal members') ethnocentric evaluations.

The first subsection highlights the significance of social process when arriving at a conception of 'physical perfection' which is stigmatising in non-participants' eyes. It shows that bodybuilding and mainstream evaluations of bodily perfection digress, and that 'extreme' muscularity is denigrated outside the subculture (Aoki 1996: 67). Since muscles are typically equated with masculinity, this issue is well documented for female physique bodybuilders who transgress the sex/gender system (e.g. Mansfield and McGinn 1993, Schulze 1990). However, as noted in Chapter 2, male bodybuilders may also transcend normative (i.e. widely accepted) bodily limits to the extent that they evoke feelings of repulsion and disgust (St Martin and Gavey 1996: 47). Overly muscular male bodybuilders may not lose their masculinity in the same way that female bodybuilders lose their femininity, but they too are considered grotesque by those outside the subculture (Lowe 1998: 85). Consequently, because the *types of* 'muscular body' to which 'hard-core' bodybuilders orient themselves and the types of 'muscular body' non-members tolerate are different, ongoing commitment to muscle-building entails a social process of becoming. During this process the individual learns to define 'Sizeably Muscular and Exceptionally Lean Bodybuilding Physiques' as aesthetically pleasing.

This aspect of bodybuilding ethnophysiology is less important for individuals striving to create 'Moderately Muscular and Typically Fairly Lean Bodies'. Following the 1980s fitness boom, these 'Athletically Muscular/Toned Bodies' are widely endorsed outside bodybuilding subculture. (See Glassner, 1990, on the representational significance of the 'fit-looking' body.) While social process therefore seems unimportant, this does not invalidate the general argument for two main reasons.

First, the exercised and dieted body is prescribed and valorised within our larger society *only up to a certain point*. As muscle mass increases and body-fat decreases, the more outlandish it becomes and thus (depending upon the individual's previous contact with bodybuilding subculture) the greater the significance of an acquired appreciation. Second, bodybuilding ethnophysiology entails more than simply admiring the superficiality of the specular body. In shaping members' perceptions, this schema provides an understanding of the ascetic commitment necessary to accrue substantial muscularity. This quasi-religious awareness renders types of bodybuilding physique more or less impressive to subcultural aesthetes.

The first subsection establishes that indigenous and non-bodybuilding conceptions of physical perfection digress (at some juncture). The second subsection then underscores the process of *acquiring an ethnophysiological appreciation*. Since favourable perceptions of the 'abnormal, extreme and unattractive body-building body' (Aoki 1996: 67) are temporally contingent and are learnt in the subcultural context, individual commitment to the 'risky' practice of bodybuilding *could* be independent of antecedent predispositions, viz. a masculinity-in-crisis within the larger society, feelings of inadequacy and a wish to embody the physical trappings of hegemonic masculinity.

Finally, bodybuilders – who are both in and of the larger society – recognise 'Sizeably Muscular Bodies' may be the focus of 'incivil attention' (Smith 1997). Although participants learn to view 'outlandish' bodies as more or less 'impressive', sensitivity to actual or potential negativity may check their wish to attain or maintain 'excessive' muscularity. This recognition of culturally normative standards, that is, members' acknowledged risk of being stigmatised outside of the subculture, is particularly relevant and is broached in both subsections.

BODYBUILDING, DRUGS AND RISK

From frog to impressive bodybuilding physiques

Bodybuilding physiques and 'fit-looking' bodies are not radically dissimilar. The former are an extension and exaggeration of the latter. However, while body-builders' normative standards interpenetrate with larger societal values, if one sufficiently extends and accentuates any values then at some juncture they must become different values (Taylor *et al.* 1973: 187). Certainly for the out-group (non-bodybuilders), 'marginal members' (fitness orientated weight trainers), and 'bodybuilders' sharing an affinity for body-sculpting as opposed to building, the aesthetic criteria of 'successful' physique bodybuilding are different from their own. One trainer interested in 'body-sculpting', for example, told me that the accomplished bodybuilder's physique (understood here as a singular concept) is not aesthetically pleasing from his perspective:

Noel: If you take the bodybuilding too far you can look like a frog, and who wants to look like a frog?

LM: What do you mean, 'a frog'?

Noel: ... Mmmm, well, if you can imagine getting hold of a frog by its front legs and holding it up, and looking at it from behind. You've got the big back like the bodybuilder spreading his lats [latisimus dorsi], the small waist and the big thighs.

(Field Diary: 27 August 1994)

While interviewing Noel I asked him to elaborate this remark after he claimed it is possible to become 'too muscular'. The extract is noteworthy for three main reasons. First, it highlights how social process renders many gym members willing and able to accrue 'excessive' muscularity. Second, it suggests perceptions of muscular bodies are relative and context bound. And third, the unflattering similes employed to describe the type of physique displayed by accomplished male bodybuilders are particularly colourful and are indicative of his value-orientation:

Noel: That's where you've gone to the extreme. I mean, once they've got to that size it's competition within the gym. They go into it to be bigger than the next bodybuilder next to them, as much or more than him [...] and before they know it with the years of bodybuilding they've increased and the comparison in the gym is not as great [i.e. the differences between the levels of muscularity are subtle in this context as judged by non-bodybuilders] because they're all the same size and they're competing to get bigger all the time. They're feeling good in that gym: 'sure I feel great, look good'. When they put their clothes on they're not too bad. When they walk into a pub then, they just know that they're big lads, and it looks good in clothes, big lads. But as soon as it comes to the beach they get a shock I think. I've seen it many a time. They go onto that beach and they look bloody big and all of a sudden they realise that all eyes on them are not swooning ... you can see some girls going 'ugh!' You do see it, 'ugh!' They wouldn't say it to your face, but you know that's what the expressions are on people's faces. You only have to walk past and in the corner of your eye you can see someone going 'ugh!' And that's a typical person who's not got a body like that that says that. At the end of the day that [look] has gone too far and they don't look athletic anymore. You put Linford Christie walking past, and they'll all swoon, and Linford Christie's a fine physique of what a male ...

LM: The body-beautiful yeah?

Noel: Yeah, you know, it's muscular, it's lean, it's a tiger isn't it? A puma, compared to a rhinoceros.

LM: So you would compare a bodybuilder to a rhino then? [...] I know you've compared them to a frog.

Noel: A frog or a rhino and Linford Christie is a puma. [Noel went on to talk about how height is an intervening variable. For him, tall bodybuilders carry muscle better.] You normally find the average height of a bodybuilder is 5'6'', 7, 8 [...] so they go onto the beach with a physique like bloody that wide as well, they're like an Oxo cube. Do you know what I mean?

(Interview: Respondent 3)

What is impressive according to one aesthetic code is not necessarily appealing from another. This point is also evidenced below where indigenous and ethnocentric evaluations are counterbalanced by the same individual. Soccer offered a particularly graphic description of a fellow bodybuilder who was 'probably awesome from a bodybuilding point of view' but who would be considered 'ridiculous' by the mainstream public. While such ambivalence and oscillation of identification are important considerations in relation to stigma and its management (Goffman 1968: 130), Soccer's reference to non-Western body modification practices and ethnophysiological perceptions of physical beauty is particularly appropriate here (similarly, see Brain 1979):

Soccer told me about Grim Reaper whom he recently saw in the supermarket.

Soccer: He's fucking massive. When I say massive I mean he's taken it to the point where it's fucking ridiculous. He was just a one man freak show. You know where you can take the bodybuilding to the point where it's not seen as acceptable? Well, he'd taken it one stage beyond that. He couldn't even walk properly, he walked like this [hunching his shoulders up and waddling], like a fucking clockwork toy. If you asked 99 per cent of the population what they thought about the way he looked then they'd say ridiculous. He probably thinks he looks attractive but I bet no one else does. Like, you get these African tribes where they put these discs in their mouth and ears. They do that because they think it looks attractive and in their eyes it is. Well, I'd say it was the same with this bloke. He thinks he looks good but he doesn't. I suppose to the average person on the street there's no difference between him and a 30 stone Mr Blobby fat man. If you asked them which they preferred then they'd probably have to flick a coin to decide.

LM: It's unusual in that you've trained for years and yet you describe him in this way. I thought that you'd be more likely to say he looked impressive rather than ridiculous.

Soccer: Don't get me wrong. From a bodybuilding point of view he's probably awesome. I don't know for sure though as he was fully dressed. He might be bloated [suffering oedema due to excessive steroid use] or he might actually have a very impressive physique. If he took his top off then I might change my mind about how he looked, and I'd be the first to say he's got a good physique. He might look like Dorian Yates with his top off. I don't know. But in clothes, and to the average person on the street he looks fucking stupid. No different than a big fat man.

(Field Diary, 11 March 1995: Olympia Gym)

Despite (or in spite of) their sheer size, bodybuilders may be ridiculed when interacting with 'normals'. The following extract, solicited from an elite physique competitor, is illustrative. It is recognised, of course, that these accounts lend themselves to the type of conversation analysis undertaken by Widdicombe and Wooffitt (1995: 116–36). Similar to punks, bodybuilders do 'being ordinary' (Sacks 1984; cited by Widdicombe and Wooffit 1995: 119) when complaining about negative assessments. However, such data also inform us that accomplished bodybuilders – though personally satisfied with their bodies – may use clothing as a technique of information control (Goffman 1968) in public settings sanctioning partial nudity. This, in turn, serves as a strategy for deflecting the unappreciative attention of non-participants:

Alan: I am satisfied with the way my body looks, it's just that I don't think other people [the public] appreciate it. They don't appreciate the work that I put into it. OK I've taken steroids – they say 'yeah, you're a steroid freak'.

But they don't realise the work I've also had to put in to develop it. The prime example is, we went to the beach a couple of years back and it was just before I did the [Mr.] Universe, and I was in a pair of shorts and there were five young women, if you like, around the twenty mark, four of them reasonable – one of them really, really grossly overweight. She was the one that passed the comment! We were with friends, with family and friends – she made comments loud enough for everybody to hear, that she thought I was grossly-overdeveloped, I looked sick, disgusting, you know [...] Normally I just shut myself off to it, but now I won't even put a pair of shorts on or whatever. I'll go on the beach and I'll be like this [wearing clothes]. And it's not that I'm not satisfied with my own body, it's the fact that I don't feel I'm appreciated. I think in a lot of people's eyes outside of bodybuilding I'm a bit of a freak.

LM: I'd have thought such a reaction would have been strange today. I mean you have the ideal of what the body should look like – low fat and muscular.

Alan: Yeah, I think it's more the athletic type of physique though. Bodybuilding takes the athletic physique one stage further, and for some people that's too freaky.

(Field Diary, 26 January 1995: Al's Gym)

The mesomorph may be a masculinist cultural ideal (Klein 1993: 242), provided this body-image equals 'Moderately Muscular and Typically Fairly Lean Bodies'. However, the aesthetics of 'Sizeably Muscular and Exceptionally Lean Bodies' must be learnt in the subcultural context if the individual is to 'embrace this profane religion of physicality that is bodybuilding' (Wacquant 1995b: 163). As stated by Becker (1963: 56): 'what was once frightening and distasteful becomes, after a taste for it is built up, pleasant, desired, and sought after'. Rod, who developed his physique to the extent that it secured him a national title, had the following to say (though as a qualification, while this bodybuilder *thought* he wanted to display his 'new' body at the beach, this was something he had not yet done):

Rod: Now I've been using a bit of gear [steroids] I know what's going to happen this year. I'll walk onto the beach and they'll go 'Jesus Christ, he's a bodybuilder!' And I never would have got that without steroids, and to be honest, a lot of people would say 'well, I really don't want to look like that, I don't want to be like that', and in one sense I never used to, but once you start seeing yourself in the mirror and you start seeing the body take shape, you think you can't wait to get down to that bloody beach and rip your top off and say 'look at this!'

(Interview: Respondent 18)

BODYBUILDING, DRUGS AND RISK

Acquiring an ethnophysiological appreciation

Undoubtedly the functionality of talk is an important analytic concern: the following excerpts, for example, may be considered 'techniques of neutralisation' (Sykes and Matza 1957) or rhetorical devices which negate the questionable features of bodybuilding. (See also Edwards and Potter, 1992, on the rhetorical use of language.) However, these accounts – voiced by bodybuilders who had competed at the local level – also inform us about their subcultural perceptions which serve to structure and maintain their 'deviant' activities over time. In short, they highlight what is, in effect, a necessary condition for ongoing muscular enhancement, viz. an acquired ethnophysiological appreciation:

Ken: My legs, you put them next to a normal person, and they wouldn't even know what they were. And it's only since I've been a bodybuilder I've realised how different a set of legs can look from a bodybuilder to a normal person. You know, bloody hell, there's nothing to a normal person's legs! I've got tear drops [muscle located on the inside leg just above the knee], I've got splits [separation between muscles], I've got lines everywhere in my legs and it's a hell of a difference, like you know.

(Interview: Respondent 43)

Doug: The World's Strongest Man, you can see the different types of muscle mass. I can look at their muscle mass and say 'yeah, that's for that purpose'. The same with weight lifters. The same with bodybuilders. You can identify between, you know, different types of muscle mass. Watch the 'World's Strongest Man'. People say 'oh, he's a big bugger isn't he? Huge, big arms'. But no definition. You know? It's all there for strength and power. We can identify what it's there for and the people who don't train can't. 'Why isn't he a bodybuilder? Look at him, why isn't he?' But we can tell the difference, because we're involved in it.

(Interview: Respondent 29)

Similarly, consider the following exchange. Again this points towards the temporal nature of social action and the importance of acquired ethnophysiology during the career of the bodybuilder:

LM: Is this [body] image [which you have in mind and which you aspire to build] any different from the one you initially had when beginning weight-training?

Tony: Oh yes, it has changed. If I was to imagine if I was to look like I do now when I was doing it [in the beginning] I would have probably thought I would have been happy. But you obviously want to get bigger all the time. When I first started off I really didn't know much about body types as I do now. You know? What would be lacking. Things like rear delts, rear delts missing [...] To the ordinary person they don't really notice. If you see someone who has got a bit of muscle, a big chest you just think he is muscular. They [non-bodybuilders] don't notice a big chest, more shoulder, they don't notice that.

(Interview: Respondent 4)

These narrators' self-reflexive awareness that their aesthetic taste has been cultivated in the bodybuilding *habitus* is unsurprising given mainstream negativity, and is an interesting contrast to Bourdieu *et al.*'s (1991: 108) claim that 'the love of art is loath to acknowledge its origins'. More importantly, such data support Wacquant's observation that participation in bodybuilding progressively transforms 'the mental and corporeal schemata through which the individual perceives reality and endows it with meaning and value' (1995b: 173). For non-affiliative members perception is increasingly indeterminate and is proportionately related to the social distance between the individual and bodybuilding subculture. In the absence of bodybuilding ethnophysiology, onlookers may mistake muscle for fat. Soccer, whose body-fat composition was measured using skin-fold callipers at around 10 per cent, and who was thus not fat by non-bodybuilding standards (*cf.* McArdle *et al.* 1986), said:

Soccer: ... my flat mate, Wayne, had arranged to meet these two women opposite the night-club where I was working [as a doorman]. One of the women who passed the night-club said to Wayne 'was that your mate on the doors, the big fat one'. Wayne goes 'he's on the doors, yeah, but he's not fat, there's not an ounce of fat on him, he's a bodybuilder'. She just said 'well, he looks fat to me'. [...] It's strange but if you don't know what you're looking for I suppose as a bodybuilder you can look fat to ordinary people. I was on the beach once and there was this bodybuilder walking along. I overheard two women talking behind me. They said 'Oooow, look at him. Is that muscle or fat?' And the thing is, this bloke had a terrific physique. He wasn't fat at all.

(Field Diary, 8 October 1994: Pumping Iron Gym)

Although, as indicated above, accomplished (stigmatised) bodybuilders may feel uncomfortable when subjected to the public gaze, it is not contradictory to exhibit the physique in contexts occupied by those who have acquired an ethnophysio-logical appreciation. Bodybuilding competitions, for example, are social fields where developed bodies are seen to possess symbolic value and are positively acknowledged (*cf.* Shilling 1993: 127):

Sonny: I wouldn't go to a swimming baths and things like that, you know, because I didn't want people looking and all that. I used to be covered and you know […] I trained to get on well in bodybuilding […] I just didn't want to sort of show it off like, only in the right place.

LM: You didn't want to be looked at?

Sonny: Yes, I get embarrassed everybody stopping and having a look, and I didn't want all that.

LM: I suppose on stage when you're competing everyone's still looking at you.

Sonny: Yeah, but that's the reason you do it. You do it for that day, for that competition. You want to win that competition. You know? That's your goal isn't it?

(Interview: Respondent 17)

Displaying 'excessive' muscularity outside the subculture, and the attendant risk of being subject to breaches of the 'civil inattention' rule (Goffman 1963), often entails adopting an air of defiance or indifference. Again, several of my informants were aware that muscle read according to acquired ethnophysiological criteria differs from non-members' evaluations:

Soccer: Because I'm out of shape at the moment I feel I can walk around without a shirt [on a sunny day like today] because I'm more like a normal person now. I'm not to the extreme where people look and, from their expressions, are saying 'that muscle is just too much. He's gone too far'.

Mick [a national junior champion]: I was like that. I'd wear sweatshirts and stuff in the summer. I don't give a shit now.

Soccer: Yeah, well, I think I need to adopt that attitude. Unfortunately I don't like it when I get that reaction 'what the fuck?' At the moment it's OK as I look less freaky to people on the street. I should have the same attitude as you though Mike. I should say 'this is my body, this is the way I want to look, so if you don't like it then fuck it. I don't give a shit'. I do give a shit though.

(Field Diary, 2 August 1995: Pumping Iron Gym)

Social process, variable definitions of 'the perfect body', and the balancing of indigenous and mainstream perspectives during the career of the bodybuilder are themes clearly illustrated by Soccer. This bodybuilder for over twenty years, who remarked that he initially started training 'to sort of build up my physique a little bit' experienced ongoing conflict vis-à-vis what he had learnt to see as impressive from an insiders' perspective and what he believed outsiders' (or, more specifically, heterosexual women) considered a 'body beautiful'. After peaking at a muscular body weight of 16½ stone, Soccer felt he transgressed mainstream limits during a Summer holiday; here 'I read from people's eyes that they thought I'd taken it too far. That I'd ruined a good physique by going overboard with the bodybuilding' (Field Diary, 19 September 1994). Of course, developed muscularity is similar to primitive body decoration, painting and masking in that it represents a reversible form of body-marking (Falk 1995: 98). Less than one year later, and 12 pounds lighter, Soccer believed he had 'put things into perspective' and settled for a type of physique which he previously considered inferior from a bodybuilding point of view:

Soccer: At the end of the day I just want a body beautiful which is impressive to the average person on the street. To someone like Alan, who has a trained eye, there'll be flaws in my physique. A bodybuilding judge may say to me: 'Yeah, you've got a good foundation but you need to work on this, this and that'. Well, I couldn't give a fuck what a bodybuilding judge would say. If I was good in his eyes I'm pretty sure the average woman on the street would think I'm fucking disgusting because to be good in a body-building judge's eyes you have to look like a freak, especially today in the 1990s. I don't want to look like a competitive bodybuilder, I'm not gonna compete. No, I want what is considered a sexy physique like a Chippendale. Now, if a Chippendale entered a bodybuilding show they'd get pissed all over [beaten]. A Chippendale wouldn't really stand a chance. Even so, I bet 98 per cent of the population would agree that a Chippendale physique is far more pleasing to the eye than Dorian Yates. Whereas bodybuilders who are no more than 2 per cent of the population would rate Dorian Yates. Now, you have to decide what you want to aim for, but personally I'll go with 98 per cent who say the Chippendale has got the best physique.
(Field Diary, 19 March 1995: Olympia Gym)

In sum, there are different evaluations of 'the muscular body (bodies)' which is itself a variable project. Individuals wishing to create a type of 'Sizeably Muscular' physique – and who thus risk social stigmatisation – must adopt a certain pers-pective which is *acquired through a social process of becoming*. Participants sensitive to actual or potential negativity may readjust their ethnophysiologically informed preferences and aim to develop or maintain a type of muscular body which is a closer physical approximation to hegemonic masculinity or normative standards of beauty. Body-projects are variable: they are spatially and temporally contingent, and are increasingly dependent upon bodybuilding ethnophysiology the further muscle transgresses mainstream normative limits. This argument, which is applicable to men even though 'muscle' is widely considered a 'natural' aspect of masculine appearance, may be safely assumed to extend to female bodybuilders who are threatening to a femininity conceived in terms of frailty. Indeed, bodybuilding ethnophysiology acquires greater significance given the power of the sex/gender system in constraining women's interactions with new body technologies (Balsamo 1996).

Conclusion

Bodybuilding lends itself to various different readings within and outside the academe. Although questioning the generality of existing knowledge claims, I am therefore not dismissing the argument that muscle may figure in the construction of masculine identity and the reassertion of hegemonic masculinity. 'The muscular body' may be abstracted from embodied culture and recast as a singular concept which is, among many other things, the literal embodiment of patriarchal power (White and Gillett 1994). Bodybuilders, who are capable of homogenising body-projects through a process of 'carnal reflexivity' (Crossley 1995), may support the claim that 'the muscular body' valorises a dominance based notion of masculinity which naturalises male privilege. This may contribute to the attraction of bodybuilding, either in the presence or absence of primitive psychic anxiety attributable to early life experiences (*cf.* Jefferson 1998: 94). And, at the level of abstracted affinities 'muscle' signifies potentially violent masculinity (Mansfield and McGinn 1993: 50) rendering some willing to try the style of the bodybuilder. This *aspect* may also contribute to the sustainability of bodybuilding, drug-taking and other risk behaviours. For example, bodybuilders working as 'bouncers' – in subordinating the (feminine?) aesthetics of the 'body beautiful' to the display of menace (Jefferson 1998) – derive income and a sense of masculinity from their bodily capital.

Undoubtedly, muscular bodies are heavily gendered and may be central to an individual's identification as a man (Jefferson 1998: 78). Commenting upon the feminisation of American culture towards the end of the nineteenth century and the emergence of a visible gay subculture, Kimmel (1994) describes the importance of 'pumping up' to many men anxious to demarcate themselves from women and effeminate gay men. The cultural relationship between muscularity and masculinity invariably means that female bodybuilders often have to negotiate powerful gendered discourses if they are to construct 'excessive' muscularity and preserve a secure (hetero)sexual feminine identity (Lowe 1998). However, and without downplaying the significance of the sex/gender system, centrally this chapter argued that the 'masculinist imagery' of 'the muscular body' alongside feelings of gender and personal insecurity are neither necessary nor sufficient conditions for bodybuilding. From those data reported here, it could be argued that in the sport and art of bodybuilding, commitment is dependent upon a 'pictorial competence' learnt through habit and exercise (Bourdieu *et al.* 1991: 109). Correspondingly, personal involvement in 1990s physique bodybuilding (and associated 'risky' practices) could be independent of *antecedent* anxieties caused by a masculinity-in-crisis in the larger society.

Three final points. First, additional data support this chapter's central argument. Documenting spatial variations in perception, where male respondents assess photographs of different types of muscular body, underscores the importance of acquired ethnophysiology among today's bodybuilders. In contrast to hard-core bodybuilders (and other affiliative members e.g. bodybuilding judges), weight trainers on the 'margins' of the group could not offer an 'artistic deciphering' of 'Sizeably Muscular and Exceptionally Lean Competition Standard Bodybuilding Physiques'. In the absence of bodybuilding ethnophysiology they disparaged 'excessively' muscular bodies, personally constructed moderately muscular bodies (physically approximating hegemonic masculinity) and rejected steroids (Monaghan 2001).

Second, in focusing upon bodybuilding ethnophysiology I am not appealing to a single element as an explanation (Silverman 1993). Within postmodernity or visually oriented consumer culture, reasons for technologically refashioning the body are manifold. Following Featherstone (1991) and Glassner (1990), reasons for bodywork extend beyond the perceived vanity and insecurity characteristic of superficial ornamental culture (Faludi 1999). Even 'transgressive' bodybuilders may invoke the importance of 'the look' and position themselves within culturally 'familiar discursive and representational space' (Schulze 1990, see also Crossley 1995: 51 on how we can study 'the body as a being which constructs representations of itself – or of other bodies'). Through a retrospective glance, 'because motives' (Schutz 1967) may be voiced by participants, including their wish to signify fe/male positive attributes such as health, youth, social status and sexual attractiveness. While some feminists interpret this to mean gym-bred men have been objectified, 'feminised' and are ultimately 'in crisis' (Faludi 1999: 40), an alternative gender-wide reading suggests bodybuilders are 'fit for postmodern self-hood' (Glassner 1990).

Finally, it is worth stressing that the body exists both as a sentient and a sensible being (Crossley 1995: 46). Accordingly, the sensuous experiences associated with training, for example, – the so-called 'erotics of the gym' (Mansfield and McGinn 1993: 66) which bodybuilders 'learn to enjoy' – further contribute to the attraction of bodywork. Interestingly, the redefinition and experience of self-induced, controllable and non-injurious 'pain' as wholly constructive contrasts with many other masculinist sports where the body is simultaneously a weapon and target for violence (Young *et al.* 1994: 184). Moreover, the learnt capacity to convert non-injurious pain to pleasure contributes to the sustainability of bodybuilding. This necessary condition for bodybuilding may also be independent of personal and gender inadequacy and the wish to embody hegemonic masculinity.

The subject of drug-taking in bodybuilding, which Klein (1995) attributes to constructs of personal/gender inadequacy and the abandonment of health, is detailed in the next two chapters. Undoubtedly, hegemonic masculinity would seem to mesh well with the features of masculinity that are seen as negative to health (Annandale 1998: 140). However, drug use (as opposed to abuse) in bodybuilding – instrumental in creating 'perfect bodies' – is conducted within ethno-pharmacological parameters aimed at minimising harm while maximising benefits. Thus, while side effects (which could be considered relatively harmless but undesirable) are often reported by steroid users (Korkia and Stimson 1993: 89–94), many steroid-using bodybuilders are able to resist the claim that they are voluntarily risk-inducing because of their 'irresponsible' actions. Adopting a calculative orientation to risk behaviour, many claim they carefully manage serious and cumulative steroid risks by conducting use within generalised and flexible ethno-pharmacological parameters.

Chapter 5

Bodybuilding ethnopharmacology: managing steroid risks

The following excerpt, which constructs steroid users as responsible for the surveillance and management of their own risk environment, was taken from a bodybuilding steroid handbook. As well as accepting diverse information sources within 'risk society' (Beck 1992, Giddens 1991), a calculative orientation to risk behaviour is espoused by the bodybuilding author:

> There just doesn't seem to be any room for ignorance if an athlete has decided to use steroids. Any and all information must be applied in an effort to maintain a therapeutic course; one which is centred on getting maximum benefits while confronting the fewest side effects. In the risky business of self administering anabolic steroids, a layman's [*sic*] knowledge just isn't enough.

> (Phillips 1991: 9)

According to ethnographic work undertaken in the USA, the pharmacological knowledge possessed by experienced steroid-using bodybuilders is sophisticated (Augé and Augé 1999, Goldstein 1990). Similarly, qualitative research in the UK suggests that many bodybuilders' knowledge of steroid ingredients, effects, side effects and regimens, qualifies them as 'ethnopharmacologists' (Korkia and Stimson 1993: 122). That is, 'lay' people with a detailed subcultural understanding of the pharmacological properties of particular compounds, consisting of a taxonomy of different steroids, dosages, administration routes and complex cycling theory (Bloor *et al.* 1998). Of course, variability exists in the social distribution of ethnopharmacological knowledge: the stock of *actual* knowledge at hand differs from one individual to the next (Schutz 1967: 14). However, the mere existence of this knowledge, crystallised in steroid handbooks and readily accessible to bodybuilders, enables many to present themselves and/or their drug-using peers as competent risk managers. An invaluable counterweight, one could argue, to the pathological view of risk-taking which sees risk behaviour as merely irrational (Bloor 1995: 22).

This chapter describes the ethnopharmacology of steroid use in bodybuilding. Predicated on the assumption that the material world (including the materiality of the body) is rational, predictable, and amenable to human control, this 'indigenous' knowledge is aimed at maximising benefits while limiting drug-related harm. To be sure, bodybuilders choosing to use steroids, similar to surgeons choosing to work with patients others see as 'high risk' (Fox 1998: 680), may reject the judgement that their behaviour is risky. Also, bodybuilders' risk activities may remain largely unconsidered or habitual rather than calculative (Bloor 1995: 98–100). Nevertheless, if steroids are ascribed hazardous characteristics (certain types are deemed more hazardous than others), then bodybuilding ethnopharmacologists consider themselves capable of managing the possible/identifiable/knowable dangers of chemically constructing the physical body. In the process of transformation or 'becoming other' (Fox 1998: 678) bodybuilding ethnopharmacology serves to establish many bodybuilders (at least within their minds) as responsible by reducing drug side effects and the doubt and uncertainty which risk-taking could generate at a cognitive level.

Empirical materials are reported and analysed under four main headings: bodybuilding steroid classification, steroid cycle theories, experimental investigation and the social distribution of ethnopharmacological knowledge. Here a taxonomy of steroids is presented, parameters for 'correct' usage are noted, the variability of steroid use is highlighted and likely ethnopharmacological candidates are identified. Recognising the uses and limitations of cultural theory (Bellaby 1990), this chapter documents the role of group in shaping risk acceptability among bodybuilders as well as diversity in steroid-related risk behaviour.

Bodybuilding steroid classification

General principles of taxonomic analysis

The perceived costs and benefits of taking steroids, either alone or in combination, depends upon the ascription of hazardous characteristics to different types of steroid. Bodybuilders' ethnopharmacological stock-of-knowledge, which instructs participants how to see steroids, how to differentiate between them, thereby providing the means by which to engage with the world, is partly analysable in terms of taxonomy and nomenclature. That is, the systematic naming and classification of different types of steroid.

Ethnographers have furthered understanding of indigenous cosmology through taxonomic analysis (Spradley 1979). A basic premise of such analyses is that people manage their affairs by aggregating, differentiating and classifying objects and events. Social life is dependent upon the human capacity to recognise similarities and differences and to mark these similarities and differences linguistically. A necessary precondition for understanding and acting is the ability to isolate linguistically recognised groupings of objects of varying degrees of inclusiveness. These classes may be referred to as 'taxa' which may be subjected to taxonomic analysis.

Medical anthropologists have conducted taxonomic analyses. Frake (1980), for example, has conducted a taxonomic analysis of 186 'disease names' among the Subanun of Mindanao. Frake first explains that categories are frequently inclusive of others, are superordinate and operate at a less specific level of contrast, by providing a taxonomic hierarchy where the category 'dog' is taken as the object of analysis (1980: 109–10). Thus, in moving from the specific to the general, there are, for example, poodles (which are contrasted with, say, collies), dogs (which contrast with cats), animals (which contrast with plants). In their turn, dogs as particular types of animal also belong to the zoologically sophisticated superordinate categories 'canine', 'mammal', 'vertebrate'. Frake (1980: 110) explains that a taxonomic hierarchy comprises different sets of contrasting categories at successive levels, the categories at any one level being included in a category at the next higher level. He adds: 'taxonomies divide phenomena into two dimensions: a horizontal one of discrimination (poodle, collie, terrier) and a vertical one of generalization (poodle, dog, animal)' (Frake 1980: 110).

A taxonomic hierarchy of types of steroid

Drug researchers have already identified some of the more popular types of illicitly used steroids (Evans 1997). However, this information has not been documented in relation to bodybuilders' subcultural classificatory system. In identifying some of the many different types of steroid used by bodybuilders, Table 5.1 provides an ethnopharmacological taxonomy. This information is partial. For example, mention is made to some, rather than all, pharmaceutical companies producing specific

Table 5.1 An ethnopharmacological taxonomy of different steroids used in bodybuilding

STEROIDS (Gear, 'Roid's or Stuff)

THE ANABOLICS (Safe Steroids, Cutting Gear, Hardeners or Lean Builders)

ORAL ANABOLICS (tablets and capsules)			INJECTABLE ANABOLICS (intramuscular)	
			OIL-BASED LONGER-LASTING	WATER-BASED SHORT-LASTING & FAST-ACTING
Stanozolol (Winstrol)	Methenolone (Primobolan)	Oxandrolone (Anavar)	Nandrolone Decanoate (Deca-Durabolin)	Stanozolol (Winstrol Depot)
Winstrol			Decadurabolin by Organon / Deca by Organon / Primobolan Depot	Primobolan Acetate

THE ANDROGENICS (The Testosterones, Nasties, Mass Steroids, Bulking Gear or Builders)

ORAL ANDROGENICS (tablets and capsules)						INJECTABLE ANDROGENICS (intramuscular)			
						OIL-BASED LONGER-LASTING		SHORT-LASTING & FAST-ACTING	WATER-BASED
Oxymetholone	Fluoxymesterone (Halotestin)	Methandrostenolone (Dianabol)	Methandione	Testosterone Undecanoate	Sustanon 250	Testosterone Cypionate	Testosterone Enanthate	Testosterone Propionate	Testosterone Aqueous Suspension
Anadrol / Anapolon 50		Buit WRG / Russian Dianabol / Dianabol	Anabol & G / Pronabol / Pink Stars	Andriol / Restandol AAAR	Organon Durateston / Sustanon Omnadren ROO		Viron / Primobarol / Testoviron Propionabol VTT	Testex 250 / Virormone 100	

steroids and no attempt is made to list the amount of active ingredients contained in each product. Furthermore, native taxonomic hair-splitters could modify the diagram by including additional types and subtypes. For instance, a distinction could be drawn between veterinarian and non-veterinarian steroids. Although omitted from the table, brief reference is made to veterinarian steroids below.

On the taxonomic hierarchy, superordinate categories stand above their subordinates. The structure of the diagram is such that higher taxa are more general and inclusive than all subsequent lower level taxa which become increasingly specific and exclusive. Thus, the superordinate category 'steroids' represents the most general and inclusive taxa and may be taken in bodybuilding nomenclature as a cover term for different types of '*gear*'. (Alternative lexemes or slang diminutives are also noted.)

At the very lowest level of the taxonomy are the names of specific steroids e.g. '*Deca*' by Organon and Anapolon 50 (sometimes abbreviated to '*Napolon*'). These specific drugs belong to more generic categories which are superordinate and which are therefore read vertically. Continuing with the previous examples, these compounds respectively contain the generic pharmaceutical substance Nandrolone Decanoate (also known to bodybuilders by the specific proprietary name Deca-Durabolin) and '*Oxy's*' (Oxymetholone). In reading the taxonomy vertically upwards, Nandrolone Decanoate is classed as a '*longer-lasting, oil-based, injectable anabolic*'. Oxymetholone is classed as an '*oral androgenic*'.

As noted, taxonomic hierarchies consist of a vertical dimension of generalisation, and a horizontal dimension of discrimination. Thus, in moving vertically from the cover term '*gear*' to the next subordinate level, this category is subdivided horizontally into '*the anabolics*' (also known as '*safe steroids*', '*cutters*', '*hardeners*', or '*lean builders*') and '*the androgenics*' ('*the testosterones*', '*nasties*', '*mass steroids*', '*bulkers*' or '*builders*'). The next subordinate level of the taxonomy, if read horizontally, notes that both '*the anabolics*' and '*the androgenics*' comprise two subtypes referred to as '*orals*' and '*injectables*'. Again, the vertical and horizontal dimensions of the taxonomy presents different types and subtypes. For instance, both '*injectable androgenics*' and '*injectable anabolics*' are available in '*oil-based*' and '*water-based*' preparations which differ in their characteristics (see below).

The lowest level of the taxonomy is indicative of bodybuilders' ability to discriminate horizontally between specific steroids according to their proprietary names, the name of the manufacturer and other details. Because specific steroids are often presented in labelled boxes featuring relevant product information, packaging serves as a clear objective marker for horizontal discrimination. (Steroid books and bodybuilding magazines often contain photographs of steroids.)

As noted, Table 5.1 excludes veterinarian steroids. Although for my respondents non-veterinarian steroids were more abundant, greater in variety, and more commonly used than veterinarian drugs, animal steroids should be acknowledged. This is necessary because the logic behind using veterinarian products may be seriously questioned. Klein, for example, states: 'particularly desperate and uninformed bodybuilders [use] horse hormones' (1995: 108–9). Interestingly, bodybuilding ethnopharmacology supports their usage via a sophisticated understanding of different types of chemical compound. For example, according to one steroid handbook, Equipoise (a horse steroid) stimulates quality muscle growth with relatively few side effects such as oedema (water retention) and liver damage (Grunding and Bachmann 1995: 113–14).

Elaborating the basis for steroid classification: characteristics and (side) effects

Bodybuilders' steroid classificatory system and accompanying ethnopharmacological knowledge is elaborated below, underscoring differences between 'anabolics/androgenics', 'orals/injectables' and so on. Although methods of usage are inevitably broached, these are detailed when discussing steroid 'cycle theories'.

Bodybuilders claim 'the anabolics' are of relatively low toxicity. This class of 'gear' is often used for 'lean-building' which means achieving limited but high quality muscular gains without retaining water or fat. These drugs are also used while 'cutting' (dieting). Some of these substances, such as Oxandrolone (proprietary name: Anavar), are renowned for giving the physique a 'hard look', hence the term 'hardeners'. 'Deca' is considered neither a 'hardener' nor a 'cutter' because 'muscle-blurring' water retention is a side effect associated with this drug. However, it belongs to 'the anabolics' because its anabolic to androgenic ratio is tipped in favour of the former.

As stated by Bolin (1992a: 94): 'ideologies about steroids and their effects are seen through the lens of gender and provide a narrative of biological reductionism'. Bodybuilders' (ethno)scientific characterisation of 'anabolics' and 'androgenics' is illustrative. According to medical literature, none of the steroids exhibit a complete separation of anabolic (tissue-building) from androgenic (masculinising) activity (Kochakian 1993). However, bodybuilding ethnopharmacologists maintain that 'the anabolics', relative to 'the androgenics', exert minimal masculinising effects. Correspondingly, secondary male sexual characteristics are less likely to occur with these hormones (Phillips 1991: 4).

100

Biomedical ideas concerning steroid characteristics and side effects, which, from one perspective, are complicit with the dominant gender order that seeks to constrain 'subversive' female bodybuilding (Balsamo 1996), pattern drug-taking among 'knowledgeable' female bodybuilders. Undoubtedly, *'anabolics'* are preferred by women wary of the irreversible masculinising side effects associated with steroids in general (Strauss and Yesalis 1993), and the more potent *'testosterones'* in particular. Because virilisation is constructed as problematic for women (it is deemed embarrassing rather than life threatening), and women's 'biology' renders them particularly sensitive to steroids, the risk-to-benefit ratio associated with *'androgenics'* is often considered too great. As one female Ms Physique competitor and steroid user explained, variable steroid sensitivity between the sexes means that only the uninformed or misinformed woman would use something as androgenic as Sustanon 250. This extract also supports Green's (1997a: 476) observation that females are more likely to talk about their responsibilities for others as an appropriate part of their risk assessment role:

Sally: If men take steroids they need to take at least four times the amount that women take to have a similar effect … That's why I said women don't take as much as people think they take.

LM: Not going to need to are they?

Sally: No. I'm not talking about testosterone. Any woman with any sense wouldn't take it because it's too androgenic isn't it? But they would only need to take the tiniest amount and it's straight away a foreign body.

LM: Is it two Dianabol a day and a woman has the same testosterone level as the average man?

Sally: Yeah, so you're asking for trouble. I know a girl, in Thor's Gym, who asked for advice and was given advice – not by me – not by anyone with any sense. Somebody put her on two Sustanon a week. She'd been on it for three weeks when she asked me about it. I said: 'get off it'. I said: 'you're on something heavy [strong] … Don't touch them. You will virtually change into a man and they're not reversible'.

(Interview: Respondent 19)

Male bodybuilders concerned about some of the possible side effects associated with *'androgenics'* similarly opt for milder *'gear'*. For example, particularly androgenic substances are far more likely to *'aromatise'* (convert to the female hormone oestrogen) in male users resulting in *'bitch tits'* (gynaecomastia).

Despite their perceived relative safety, *'anabolics'* are not necessarily a more suitable choice for bodybuilders. Although bodybuilders call drugs like Winstrol,

Anavar and Primobolan highly anabolic, this simply means that they are much more anabolic than androgenic (Phillips 1991: 8). *'The androgenics'* (esters of the naturally occurring male hormone testosterone), in retaining the androgenic effect of the testosterone molecule, are considered far more potent in their muscle-building effect than the 'highly anabolic' items. However, they are also considered more toxic (Grunding and Bachmann 1995: 9). This category of steroid is favoured by bodybuilders wishing to *'bulk up'* and achieve *'mass'* (become much bigger in a relatively short time-period). This gain, however, is often associated with 'muscle-blurring' water retention; hence, competition bodybuilders prone to oedema tend to limit use of these substances to the off-season.

Alan, a successful competition bodybuilder, verbalised the distinction between *'the anabolics'* and *'the androgenics'* in the following terms. Here he also introduced a commonly accepted ethnophysiological and ethnonutritional component into his theorising:

Alan: ... There are the androgenics and the anabolics. They say that black men need to take the anabolics whereas whites should take the androgenics 'cause black men have naturally higher testosterone. Of course, testosterone is both anabolic and androgenic but they [black men] are best taking steroids which are more anabolic than androgenic like Primobolan, Anavar or Winstrol. These give you the hardness whereas the testosterones are good for packing on the mass. I've only taken anabolics like Primobolan and Winstrol when preparing for a competition. These steroids are protein sparing, meaning that the body doesn't need as much protein while you're on them. The androgenics like Dianabol and the testosterones utilise protein – they feed off the protein. The anabolics are good for contest preparation as they help me maintain muscle while getting ripped [losing body-fat]. I'm not a particularly big competitor and so I can't afford to burn muscle while dieting. I've never taken any of the testosterones, but I'm going to give them a try this year. I'm going to take a year off from competing and try and get some more size. I've been told that to be of international standard I need 5 to 6 more pounds of muscle, and so using the testosterones should help.

(Field Diary, 30 January 1994: Al's Gym)

In moving vertically downwards to the more specific and exclusive categories, bodybuilding nomenclature differentiates between *'orals'* (tablets or capsules) and *'injectables'* (intramuscular injections). Steroid injections are administered directly into a muscle such as the *'glutes'* (buttocks) rather than intravenously (into a vein) or subcutaneously (under the skin).

Classification of a steroid as either '*oral*' or '*injectable*' is an important drug characteristic vis-à-vis risk and identity negotiation. Conventional ideas about licit and illicit drug use suggest tablets are a far more acceptable, and safer, means of taking pharmaceuticals. Self-injecting is considered by many people, including neophyte heroin users, a 'risk boundary': it is deemed risky because it signifies 'deterioration' and 'junkie behaviour' (Rhodes 1997: 220). For many people the common association between injections, disease and pathology, renders the act of voluntarily injecting illicitly procured substances symptomatic of individual degeneracy:

> After training with Vin we talked about steroids. He stated that although his girlfriend knew he took 'gear' she didn't like the idea of him injecting himself. He said he could understand her view, adding that if his parents found tablets in his bedroom then it wouldn't be as bad as them finding injecting equipment. He said: 'with injections they [his parents] are immediately going to think "Junkie", "AIDS" and all that shit'.
>
> (Field Diary, 6 August 1996: Olympia Gym)

Cultural ideas about illicit drug injecting function as a powerful mechanism of social control which influence drug-taking behaviour. A new convert to steroid injecting commented about his previous reluctance to inject: 'When you *first think* about injections you think "oh my God, I'm a junkie, I'm going to become a drug freak"' (Interview: Respondent 18). Understandably, many steroid users prefer tablets during the early stages of their drug-taking career, but most go on to inject steroids (Korkia and Stimson 1993). Rhodes (1997) has observed similar processes and changing risk perceptions among other drug injectors alongside the *relativity of risk*. Experienced bodybuilders, drawing from clinical knowledge (see Street *et al.* 1996), often prefer '*injectables*' to '*orals*' because they are considered less toxic. According to Sally: 'I think injectables are safer because all tablets pass through the liver, so if there is any residue, or anything harmful in them, it gets deposited in the liver. Whereas with injectables its not. It's straight into the system' (Interview: Respondent 19).

In moving to the next subordinate level on the taxonomy, there are two subtypes of '*injectable gear*'. Unless fake, all '*injectables*' contain active ingredients suspended in a liquid solution. This solution consists of either oil or water; hence, the self-explanatory lexemes '*oil-based*' and '*water-based*'. These two subtypes, in turn, differ in their characteristics and effects which become even more specific as one moves from the more generic taxa downwards.

All '*water-based gear*' is '*fast-acting and short-lasting*'. Products such as

Testosterone Aqueous Suspension and Winstrol Depot, for example, reportedly exert an effect within one to two hours, but are active only for one or two days. This necessitates more frequent injections. Winstrol Depot, for example, is often injected every other day. '*Oil-based gear*' can either have a short half-life within the body or exert a prolonged biological effect. Primobolan Acetate, for example, is deemed effective only for a few days and must be injected more often than Primobolan Depot (Phillips 1991: 49). Similarly, substances such as Testosterone Propionate are considered '*short-lasting and fast-acting*' compared to steroids such as Testosterone Enanthate (Grunding and Bachmann 1995: 288). This ethno-pharmacological knowledge patterns drug-taking among experienced bodybuilders who, contra grid/group theory's suggestions, are neither complacent about risks nor risk takers *and* are not risk averse either (Bellaby 1990: 470). Exposure to *relatively* few steroid side effects (but experiencing side effects nonetheless) is accepted because steroids are instrumental in bodybuilding:

> I talked with Freddy [a bodybuilder for over twenty years]. He told me about some of his preferences when using the androgenics: 'Propionate is in and out, which I prefer when using a testosterone as you don't get as many side effects. I don't like enanthate as it hangs around the system for two to three weeks giving the toxins a chance to build up'.
>
> (Field Diary, 4 July 1996: Olympia Gym)

Specific products are generally classed as '*short-lasting and fast-acting*' if biologically active for less than a week. Steroids effective for seven days or more are therefore termed '*longer-lasting*'. Minimising the minor but often visible short-term side effects associated with steroids such as '*testosterone enanthate*' may enable bodybuilders to claim they are offsetting the possibility of major long-term health problems.

Specific steroids may be discriminated horizontally according to the amount of active ingredients contained in each compound and associated biological potency. The relative strength of different steroids, while an obvious criterion for horizontal discrimination, also determines (side) effects. At the most exclusive and specific horizontal level of differentiation one may identify, for example, '*oral*' Stromba and Anapolon. Stromba may be differentiated from Anapolon not only along the vertical dimension but also horizontally in terms of dosage. For instance, Stromba contains 5 milligrams of steroid per tablet, whereas Anapolon contains 50 milligrams. One respondent, in describing the drug regimen of somebody whom he considered a steroid abuser, stated about the ingredients, strength and side effects of specific steroids:

Len: I knew one fella … this is true, he was taking four Sustanon a week.

LM: 1000 milligrams then?

Len: Yeah, hang on, a Virormone a day.

LM: What's that?

Len: Virormone is a propionate [fast-acting, injectable, oil-based androgenic], but it's only a 100 milligram, not 250. The Testex is 250 propionate … and on top of all that he was taking four 'Napolon [a day] which is the most toxic steroid on the market. Shit your liver out with that stuff. Do you know what I mean? It's just a killer. Most steroids are 2.5 or 5 milligram a tab, and 'Napolon is 50, each one of them.

(Interview: Respondent 23)

As well as the amount of active ingredients, potency and toxicity of specific steroids, particular products are discriminated horizontally according to other criteria. Importantly, bodybuilders differentiate between specific products (and often the generic pharmaceutical substance contained in specific steroids) according to various effects other than the drugs' physique-enhancing properties. Thus, whereas all steroids are used by bodybuilders to help create, either directly or indirectly, 'the perfect body', different steroids reportedly exhibit different characteristics:

Dennis: With Primobolan you make nice solid gains which you tend to keep [after discontinuing use]. If on a cycle I tend to take Primobolan, and also Equipoise and Deca. I take the Equipoise which is a horse-racing steroid as it is supposed to help strengthen your tendons and ligaments. You know with a lot of the gear your muscles get stronger but your tendons don't so you're more likely to get an injury. I also take Deca to lubricate the joints. I don't know whether it's my age or what but you can just get out of a chair and your knees are creaking, or you hear your wrists cracking. Deca eases that and so your training isn't affected.

(Field Diary, 9 November 1995: Olympia Gym)

In addition to specific physical (side) effects, ethnopharmacologists differentiate horizontally between different steroids according to potential mood and behavioural effects. Aggression, or the so-called 'Roid-Rage phenomenon much publicised by the popular press, is frequently posited outside bodybuilding circles as an inevitable consequence of steroid use. The supposed bodybuilding-steroids-violence connection is explored in chapter seven.

Steroid cycle theories

Bodybuilding ethnopharmacologists typically follow a regularised and systematic pattern where periods of steroid use are interspersed with periods of abstinence. While various factors pattern steroid use (e.g. availability of certain drugs, finance, variable body-projects), a 'therapeutic' regimen aimed at maximising gains while minimising potential harm is informed by *'cycling theory'*.

Aspects of *'cycling theory'* are noted both in the academic literature (e.g. Gilbert 1993) and the foregoing analysis. For example, steroid taxonomy highlights the importance of *'anabolics'* during *'cutting cycles'* and *'androgenics'* during *'bulking cycles'*. This, however, is *'cycling theory'* at its most basic. Bodybuilding vernacular provides an indication of this knowledge which has hitherto received cursory attention. Esoteric sounding keywords and steroid phrases such as *'receptor sites'*, *'receptor mapping'*, *'plateaux's'*, *'staggering* or *'phased steroid rotation'*, *'pyramiding'* and *'stacking'* suggest a need to detail the technicalities of this knowledge. These terms, pertaining to 'correct' methods of usage, are significant. They are derived from a conceptual framework employed by bodybuilders concerned with maintaining a 'therapeutic' steroid regimen.

The experimental nature of steroid ethnopharmacology is discussed after charting dominant ethnoscientific ideas concerning the 'right way to do steroids' (Goldstein 1990: 91). Although steroid regimens vary from one person to the next, and for the same individual over time, 'sensible' use is conducted within specific pre-known parameters. Personalised *'cycles'*, modified to suit the particulars of the individual, are devised and executed within a generalised framework or paradigm which, as will be noted, legitimates the seemingly idiosyncratic steroid regimens of each athlete. This point, implicit in the following two apparently contradictory statements made by bodybuilders, informs the proceeding analysis:

> Anabolic steroids have been around for a long time – they've been used by humans for almost fifty years. Steroids are, for the most part, very 'predictable'. We know what they do and don't do …
>
> (Phillips 1996: 10)

> I know of no scientific or medical research done anywhere in the world that has determined the best way to use anabolic steroids for athletic enhancement. Consequently there is an enormous amount of mystery, secrecy, trendiness, and even a bit of voodoo and hocus-pocus surrounding steroid use. Bodybuilders […] seem to be somewhat sophisticated in steroid use, but his [*sic*] is only relative to the other sports.
>
> (Duchaine 1989: 47)

Parameters for 'correct' usage

According to bodybuilding 'Steroid Guru' and self-proclaimed 'Lab Rat' Dan Duchaine (1989: 47), there is no scientific or medical research determining the best ways of using steroids for athletic enhancement (similarly, see Korkia and Stimson 1993: 121). Hence, it would seem that the non-medical use of these substances is indeed something of a dark pill alchemy (Gaines and Butler 1974: 77). However, does illicit steroid-taking simply entail 'a bit of voodoo and hocus-pocus?' The bodybuilders' ability to claim 'steroids are, for the most part, extremely "predictable"' (Phillips 1996: 10), suggests that there is a systematic and qualified basis to their shared ethnoscientific reasoning: a point hinted at by Duchaine (1989: 47) when he states bodybuilders are somewhat sophisticated in their steroid use relative to other sports people.

Following Duchaine (1989) and Phillips (1996), it could be posited that steroid 'predictability' is a function of the (relatively) sophisticated nature of bodybuilders' ethnopharmacological stock-of-knowledge. Existing research on illicit steroid use mentions this sophistication (e.g. Augé and Augé 1999), but does not detail it. Describing the bodybuilders' rationale for *'cycling gear'* goes some way towards redressing this, making explicit the basis for 'correct' steroid usage. Examining the meaning of *'receptor site'* is essential here because this forms the crux of bodybuilders' rationale for using steroids (and many steroid accessory drugs) in a cyclical fashion.

Drawing upon the biomedical model of the body, *'receptor site'* refers to specific areas within the internal cellular structure of the body which are open to the various chemical messages transmitted by steroid molecules once injected or ingested. Such sites include skeletal muscle cells, hair follicles, sebaceous glands, certain areas of the brain and certain endocrine glands (Phillips 1991: 5). The specific biochemical and physiological actions of exogenous steroids are extremely complex (Grunding and Bachman 1995: 11). And, given the practical interests of athletes, it is largely irrelevant for them to possess an expert's insight into the cellular interactions between steroid molecules, nuclear DNA (deoxyribonucleic acid) and RNA (ribonucleic acid). As Duchaine writes: 'the average athlete has no idea how, in the biochemical sense, steroids work. He [*sic*] just knows that they do indeed get the job done' (1989: 15). However, although bodybuilders as laity are governed by practical interests, the centrality of steroid use in their sport often means that successful bodybuilders need more than a simple recipe knowledge (Schutz 1964) if they are to ensure optimum physique enhancement while limiting drug-related harm.

Documenting subcultural knowledge of *'receptor sites'* is central to understanding steroid use in bodybuilding, both in terms of its sophistication and the degree of personalised experimentation. Several facets of this knowledge are identifiable, through a systematisation of members' accounts and a reading of subcultural pharmacopoeia, which relate to ideas for effective, safer and variable usage. Importantly, bodybuilders theorise that '*receptor sites*' are:

* genetically fixed but vary in quantity and distribution from one individual to the next,
* are capable only of absorbing a certain amount of steroid in a given time-period,
* downgrade during a '*cycle*' but (partially) regenerate upon cessation of use,
* possess an affinity for different types of steroid rendering different compounds more or less effective,
* are at their most receptive among those who have trained diligently for some time without chemical assistance,
* become less effective for the older athlete, and
* are extremely sensitive in women.

In delimiting the (highly flexible) parameters for 'correct' usage, each of these practically relevant points is elaborated below. To this end, reference is made to indigenous pharmacopoeia (e.g. Duchaine 1989, Grunding and Bachmann 1995, Phillips 1991), and ethnographic data obtained during fieldwork and interviews.

In clarifying the first point, consider the following extract. This observation is concordant with Duchaine's (1989: 16) statement that '*genetics*' render some people more gifted with receptor sites than others:

> One of the regulars, who had recently made some substantial muscular gains, was at the gym counter talking to Ron (gym owner). He was telling Ron, myself and Soccer, about his current steroid regimen. He claimed to be taking one injection of Testex 250 a week before switching to Primobolan and Stromba. By all accounts he had increased his [lean] body weight from 15 to 16½ stone in eight weeks without any noticeable adverse effects. Ron first laughed at the relatively small dosages which this bodybuilder was using. The gym owner then said: 'Are you a genetic freak or what? You must have receptors on top of receptors. I've taken Sustanon [250] everyday for a month. Not a lot happened. Crap! My mate was covered in spots when he took Testex'.
>
> (Field Diary, 2 July 1995: Olympia Gym)

Genetically determined differential capacities to utilise steroids is an idea invoked by bodybuilding ethnopharmacologists to explain variable steroid (side) effects.

Stated simply, individuals vary in terms of their total number of receptors and in terms of where these sites are located and concentrated (e.g. sebaceous glands, hair follicles, muscle cells). A corollary is that the risk-to-benefit ratio for using steroids is variable, rendering 'use' and 'abuse' relative concepts. Correspondingly, determining an objective, generalisable and universally applicable steroid regimen for all users is impossible given the particular and unique characteristics of each and every-*body*. The alleged 'predictability' of steroids may cultivate an attitude of complacency among bodybuilders towards familiar risks but individual variability in susceptibility represents a possible source of uncertainty (Adams 1995: 49). Ultimately, this means bodybuilding ethnopharmacologists – while delimiting general boundaries for steroid use – believe each individual user must evaluate positive effects relative to observed and potential negative effects. This position, where the onus is placed upon the user, is indicative of the increasing responsibility assumed by individuals in assessing risk (the privatisation of risk) within late modernity (Giddens 1991).

Second, bodybuilding ethnopharmacologists claim '*receptor sites*' are only capable of utilising a certain amount of steroid in a given period. So-called '*kamikaze bodybuilders*' administer extremely high dosages in order to solicit an ergogenic/physique-enhancing effect. However, the law of diminishing marginal returns means that while this is effective, it is limited. Experiential data may be taken by the steroid-using bodybuilder to support this point, which is then theorised in terms of the capacity of '*receptor sites*':

Gary: I've been carried away in the past [to the extent that I would consider myself an abuser] … Um, if so much [steroid] works really you know, if 1 millilitre of so and so works for you, three times that amount must work better. But that's one of the reasons I've come off now. I was taking so much in the end and nothing's working. You know? So I think the body can only take in so much. The steroid receptor sites can only take in so much of the steroid anyway.

(Interview: Respondent 42)

This extract also illustrates point three; namely, muscle receptors are claimed to '*down grade*' rendering '*gear*' less effective over time (Phillips 1991: 69). Side effects associated with prolonged usage, in turn, tip the risk-to-benefit ratio in favour of the former. Taking steroids cyclically, where the user ideally has a period of abstinence equalling or exceeding the time spent using steroids, therefore becomes important in order to allow receptors to (partially) recover as well as allowing the body to 'detoxify':

Luke: After the cycle I'm on now [he was using Winstrol Depot, but now he's on Sustanon] I plan on taking eight months off [the steroids], let the receptor sites recover. Then probably use Deca and Dianabol for a month, change it around with something else and then hopefully balloon out [grow].

(Field Diary, 1 August 1994: Supermarket)

Soccer: I think that if you go on a cycle for eight to ten weeks then you should have eight to ten weeks off. Some say if you're going to do it safely then you should take three months off. I think the amount of time you have off should be the same as the amount of time you're on, but some time in the year you should take three months off.

(Field Diary, 27 June 1994: Supermarket)

Because receptors '*down grade*', muscular growth is reportedly sustained and a '*plateaux*' avoided by increasing the dosage. It is common during the first few weeks of the steroid regimen to administer incremental dosages (Goldstein 1990). This, however, is only considered effective for a short time-period. As stated by Luke: 'normally after three weeks or so the receptor sites don't recognise the steroid so no matter how much you take it doesn't make a difference' (Field Dairy, 1 August 1995). As dosages are increased potential health risks also heighten. For responsible narrators these risks are deemed unacceptably high with potent steroids. Stories of 'accidents' serve as a resource for other users to create and demonstrate their own competence (Green 1997a):

Soccer: Anapolon 50s? I tell you, that stuff is strong. I know this guy who took one a day and went boom, boom [signalling with his hands a sudden growth in the leg muscles]. He said: 'Bloody hell, if one does that I'll take two!' He did and went boom, boom, boom, boom [signalling a growth of muscle in the legs, chest, arms, and shoulders]. Again, he said: 'I know, if two does that I'll take three a day'. He did for three days and collapsed.

(Field Diary, 10 May 1995: Pumping Iron Gym)

After peaking with an optimum dosage (an effective amount with no perceived negative effects), users typically '*wean off*' by tapering the amount of steroid administered (Goldstein 1990). This method reportedly allows the body to gradually readjust during the transition to 'natural training': a technique known as '*pyramiding the cycle*'.

Fourth, '*receptor sites*' reportedly have an affinity for different types of steroid rendering different compounds more or less effective. Again, this has implications for 'correct' usage:

Bill: Anapolon has got 50 milligrams and Anavar has got 2.5 milligrams. It all depends on the receptor sites for these particular steroids. Anapolon has got very limited, small receptor sites to hit which is why it needs 50 milligrams – to hit the receptor sites. Oxandrolone – Anavar – has obviously got very easy receptor sites, the receptor sites [in the body] are very open, so that less is required. This is normally the difference. People sort of think: 'oh, the stronger the better', but it's not. This is why Anapolon shouldn't be taken really because it's quite toxic. Of that sort of 50 milligrams you might hit [the receptor sites with] sort of maybe 10 or 20, but then you've got 30 milligrams wooshing around your body, looking for the way out. You know?

(Interview: Respondent 24)

Differing receptor affinities for different drugs, as well as receptor degradation, have additional implications for practising ethnopharmacologists. The down regulation or attenuation of steroid receptors, and the potential health problems associated with large dosages, prompts bodybuilders to use various logical '*cycle*' patterns which capitalise upon different receptor affinities (Phillips 1991: 9). For instance, '*staggering*' or '*phased steroid rotation*' may be practised, which involves switching to a completely different steroid compound or compounds. It is claimed that if there is a progressive loss of sensitivity of receptors to an exogenous steroid, using different compounds *sequentially* for a short time-period (from three to six weeks) results in only slight impairment of receptor functions compared to the degree of down regulation experienced if one drug was taken for a long period of time (Phillips 1991: 69):

John: So I thought I'd read up on it. Other people talk to you about it, people who know about it, like. And they say that if you do stay on the same thing for … After about six weeks, it's not going to work for you anyway, no matter what it is. 'Cause your body gets used to it. Your receptors won't accept it any more. So after it's about six weeks, you're better off changing to … Still using an anabolic, but using a different anabolic, so your body is having something different […] So that way your body [is] still going to keep growing, whereas if you do stay on the same thing for six months you're just going to have no [positive] effect at all.

(Interview: Respondent 35)

Other methods are employed given receptor degradation and different receptor affinities. For example, '*stacking*' reportedly enhances steroid effectiveness while reducing side effects. (Importantly, this technique often involves the combined use of other drugs: see Chapter 6.) '*Stacking*', which may be combined with '*staggering*' and '*pyramiding*', is considered more *effective* than using a single steroid since the different characteristics of each substance reportedly stimulates multiple receptor sites resulting in a synergistic effect. One bodybuilder, after mentioning that his favourite '*stack*' consisted of Parabolan and three other steroids, stated:

Bill: Each steroid has got its different properties, it's got different receptor sites [...] You get better effects [when stacking] you can get power – drugs that will increase your power, drugs that will keep you tight, drugs that are therapeutic to the joints, you know, and in that stack of Parabolan you had everything. That was why it's one of the best stacks.

(Interview: Respondent 24)

Bill immediately added that this was also 'one of the healthiest stacks', pointing to an additional advantage associated with this technique. If different receptors have an affinity for different steroids, and '*stacking*' exerts a synergistic effect, then bodybuilding ethnopharmacologists claim a lower total dosage including several compounds will be equally (if not more) effective than a higher dosage of just one steroid. Allegedly, the positive effects of so-called '*steroid therapy*' are optimised while minimising the risk of side effects associated with large dosages: 'There's the harm reduction method where you'll do your best to try and minimise all the [side] effects by using more than one steroid. You know? Rather than taking a large dosage of one' (Interview: Respondent 24).

Sophisticated ethnopharmacological practices may be executed in order to minimise harm and maintain drug effectiveness. However, despite various measures, receptor populations only partially regenerate. Hence, and concerning the fifth point, '*receptors*' are at their most sensitive among individuals adhering to bodybuilding for several years without chemical assistance and who have a 'natural foundation' of muscle. For novice users who have put in the 'groundwork', muscle '*receptor sites*' are considered extremely sensitive rendering their first course extremely effective. Rod, the owner of Pumping Iron Gym and non-steroid-using bodybuilder for five years, 'felt like a bloody Greek God' after his first course of Dianabol and Anavar. He commented about the perceived additive effect of diet and previous training on '*receptor site*' functions:

Rod: I would like to say this as well mind, that I don't think that the steroids would have been so effective unless I'd have sort of got myself to this sort of peak where I was at, and the same for the other boys. I've seen boys come in here [into his gym] and think: 'Oh yeah! I'll have to do that [take steroids] like'. You know? 'I've been training six weeks now'. And they've taken it and nothing at all's happened. You know? It's purely down to hard work, diet and dedication really.

LM: Yeah. You hear about people who take steroids from day one and they just train once and take it.

Rod: No, it's a waste of time. I think to be honest when you put that sort of long-term training in before you decide to take it, the receptors in your body they become more open to sort of wanting it really.

(Interview: Respondent 18)

The 'correctness' of this ethnopharmacological knowledge means that experienced bodybuilders will view non-compliant marginal members with derision. Sanctions (subcultural rules prescribing and proscribing certain behaviours) become verbalised thus functioning as a form of social control aimed at regulating use, minimising harm and maximising benefits (*cf.* Moore 1993, Zinberg 1984):

LM: Some new comers to bodybuilding take it [steroids] from day one so what are your views about that?

Mick: Absolutely ridiculous. They deserve all the problems they get. Because they haven't got a clue about training, and you don't respond well if you take it straight off.

(Interview: Respondent 22)

Finally, age and gender are relevant. Muscle receptor sensitivity reportedly diminishes among older athletes. If greater dosages are administered to compensate for this then the risks of steroid use will increase. Concerning gender, Sally's narrative presented earlier is illustrative. As part of a continuing effort to sustain the social definition of gender there is an exaggeration of difference by social practices (Connell 1987). Women's receptors are considered extremely sensitive; correspondingly, ethnopharmacologists maintain that steroid use should be confined to weaker, less toxic drugs. Weaker steroids are deemed more appropriate for women because they facilitate bodily changes that do not significantly challenge current social definitions of femininity.

Before discussing personal experimentation an important issue requires attention. Although ethnopharmacologists claim continual steroid use decreases receptor sensitivity, some bodybuilders remain on these drugs for longer than the recommended twelve week limit. Indeed, there are bodybuilders who continue their use for years – a practice which is reportedly the norm among the sport's elite (Grunding and Bachmann 1995). Of those bodybuilders interviewed for this study, uninterrupted usage for extended periods was evidenced among high level competitors ambitious to win a British or International title. Respondents 21 (Alan),

35 (John) and 46 (Stan) fell into this category. Non-competition steroid-abusing 'bodybuilders' deemed to have unimpressive physiques and who were generally regarded by fellow members as having 'psychological problems' (e.g. Grim-Reaper at Al's Gym and Meat-Loaf at Olympia) also rarely abstained from steroid-taking. Disregarding the 'on-off-on-off' rule for '*cycling*' steroids requires attention, especially in the case of successful competition bodybuilders, because this apparently contradicts the ethnoscientific wisdom outlined above.

For bodybuilders preparing for competitions, and especially those qualifying to compete at international level, continued usage is considered necessary to maintain muscularity and condition. Alan described how his usual twenty week pre-contest '*cycle*' could extend to a twelve month course:

Alan: If I went for the NABBA Wales [National Amateur Body Building Association: Mr. Wales competition, held annually, usually in March] obviously I would have started taking them [steroids] in October, November of last year to prepare for the Wales which then I wouldn't come off them, I would have had to go straight on to the Britain [...] I would have had to carry on [with the cycle]. Then it would have been another two week carry on to the European championship and then another week on to the World Championship so with all – instead of it only being the twenty week cycle it might take it up close to thirty weeks. Then you have the Universe which is roughly August/September/October so I mean we're talking – so virtually you're on them up to October, so it's virtually twelve months continual if you follow through all those competitions.

(Interview: Respondent 21)

While continuous usage is common among high level competitors, the ability of these athletes to develop increasingly muscular physiques over time does not invalidate the above ethnopharmacological parameters. In maintaining steroid effectiveness these bodybuilders employ the '*stacking*' technique and continually change their drugs sequentially. Here the user may '*cycle*' within a larger '*cycle*' with the intention of ensuring continuous and steady progress:

LM: How would you define a cycle?

John: Six weeks is, I class as a cycle and then you know another six weeks another cycle.

LM: Of something else?

John: Yeah.

LM: So you don't have a break?

John: You don't have to [...] what I do find is by changing every few weeks my body's not getting used to nothing so I'm continuously gaining all the time like.

(Interview: Respondent 35)

However, three points need to be made about continuous usage concerning effectiveness and safety (parameters for correct usage):

First, bodybuilding ethnopharmacologists claim receptor populations still downgrade. The larger *'cycle'* is not effective indefinitely. Correspondingly, if steroids are to remain effective, use must eventually be ceased thereby allowing receptor regeneration. Following a recuperative period lasting several months, effective use may then recommence:

John: I've been back on [steroids] now since Christmas last year [i.e. using for eight months]. I had nine months off before that because I wanted to get it out of my system for a while 'cause I'd done three shows [competitions] in one year and that year I was on continuously because of competing so I thought: 'come off, have a break now, let it come out of your system and let the receptors open back up and everything'.

(Interview: Respondent 35)

Second, an individual's genetically predetermined bodily potential, it is claimed, allows elite bodybuilders to take large amounts of steroids continually over extended periods in order to develop 'Sizeably Muscular Physiques':

John was training on the other side of the gym. We [myself and Soccer] were at the counter with the gym owner. Soccer made a comment about John.

Soccer: There's a lot of natural genetics there. He is fucking awesome.

Ron (looking at me in surprise): Natural genetics? What about the ten jabs [injections] of Sustanon a week and the rest?

Soccer: Oh yeah, that aside [...] What I mean by natural genetics ... he's young, and if he can achieve that in only four years [of training]. Well, that is excellent. I've been training twenty years and I look nothing like that. I bet I could take all the steroids in the world and I still wouldn't be able to achieve what he has.

(Field Diary, 2 July 1995: Olympia Gym)

The third point concerns health risks. Steroids, similar to other medical/cosmetic technologies (e.g. breast implants) are implicated in health risks (Annandale 1998: 15), but these risks are exacerbated by the search for increasing economic and/or bodily capital. Bodybuilders generally accept that continuous usage, and the necessary incremental dosages required to ensure effectiveness, poses potentially serious long-term health problems. The increasingly 'higher standards' of competition, and the need to take large amounts of drugs over prolonged periods to ensure any chance of success, deters most bodybuilders from regularly entering physique competitions:

Nigel: I used to compete as a bodybuilder. The thing is though is the amount of gear you need just to place anywhere at the local level these days. I'm not really prepared to take the risks. A few years back when I won the junior Wales I was doing a jab [one injection] a week. I doubt that I could win the Wales now doing that. Well, when I competed I qualified for the Britain and, well ... you just can't stand next to some of the English boys. They're some of the best in the world. Afterwards we talked and they're open about the gear they're doing. They asked me what I was taking and they just laughed. Some of them were doing like, three jabs a day and handfuls of tablets. They had the attitude that if you've made the decision to take gear then you should take a load or not bother. You know, I'm not saying the more gear you take the better you are. It doesn't work like that – but at the end of the day the English boys are only flesh and blood like us so why are they so much better? If you take into account that we train just as hard – live, sleep and breath bodybuilding – then it's obvious that after taking everything into account like diet, training, genetics, the only difference is the [amount of] drugs.

(Field Diary,13 August 1995:
Informal gathering at a power lifter's home)

Other bodybuilders who recognise possible long-term health risks may accept them. Ambitious competitors, similar to professional boxers, are often willing to take risks and put their bodies on the line in the pursuit of occupational success (Wacquant 1995a: 82). The first extract below is taken from an interview with John: a young individualist who, similar to pottery factory supervisors and middle management risking serious injury in pursuit of profit, had prospects of further promotion amidst fierce competition (Bellaby 1990: 471). The second statement was by Bill (an older retired competition bodybuilder) who delayed taking steroids due to potential health risks, only later to regret his procrastination:

John: They reckon the steroids are going to actually damage you but in years to come, they can't, they're not actually going to affect you now. It's only the effects in about ten years time when you're going to get maybe arthritis or bones maybe crumbling or you may have a liver disorder. 'Cause like you know, you're body can't keep taking all that […] every drug has got an effect a side effect [if you take] too much of it […]

LM: It doesn't worry you maybe a little bit?

John: I do think about it in years to come. You know? 'How long am I going to live?' Or 'when I'm 40 am I going to be in a wheelchair or something?' But like, it's what I want now, no matter what I want when I'm 40-odd like. It's what I want now.

(Interview: Respondent 35)

Bill: When you use steroids [to the extent necessary to win competitions] you really have to weigh up the pros and cons, and you might be shortening your life. You might cause problems in later life […] A sensible person would weigh up the pros and cons and I've often – in my 'I don't give a fuck' time type of attitude, I would think I have sort of justified it all by saying that I would rather be a meteor and flash brightly through the sky than be a little twinkling star for seventy years and do nothing which is a bit – dramatic, isn't it? […] I feel that if I die tomorrow that my life's been eventful if nothing else. It certainly hasn't been humdrum, and it hasn't been boring […] Bodybuilding's opened doors to me … I've done a lot of things in life. I've travelled through bodybuilding, and I've had money through bodybuilding and I've had lots of good friends through bodybuilding and I've had lots of good experiences through bodybuilding. You know? So – not that I've got a death wish but […] if I had my time again, I probably would have started taking steroids earlier, not wasted my – not so much my youth, but – if I'd taken them when I was 25 perhaps […] I would have been much more competitive than what I have been now in the last couple of years and so I might have done more in the sport.

(Interview: Respondent 24)

Bodybuilders disregarding the 'on-off-on-off' 'cycle' rule accept long-term health problems are a real possibility. No doubt, the standards aspired to by today's competition bodybuilders necessitates lengthy steroid courses – an observation which prompts some indigenous authors (e.g. Phillips 1996: 10–13) to call for a revaluation of the sport's judging criteria. However, since lengthy 'cycles' seem to be the norm among high-level competitors, and participants far exceed the performance levels of their predecessors, these drug regimens are deemed effective (Grunding and Bachmann 1995: 320). In accepting that such usage is potentially dangerous, these bodybuilders acknowledge ethnopharmacological parameters for 'correct' usage. Just as 'taking certain risks may be essential to building up social identities' (Green 1997b: 138), taking 'excessive' steroid dosages over prolonged periods may be essential to 'building up' championship standard physiques. Ignoring safety aspects, however, is personal preference rather than irrationality (Douglas and Calvez 1990).

The three points outlined above are equally relevant when considering the drug regimens of other gym members, such as non-competitors who have no aspirations of achieving professional bodybuilding stardom. Grim-Reaper, so called because his prolonged and excessive steroid use was likely to be the death of him, trained at Al's Gym. Meat-Loaf from Olympia, was another well known trainer regarded locally as a steroid abuser. Grim-Reaper, who trained for a while at Olympia, was the most talked about. From conversations with Reaper's associates and with the man himself, it emerged that he had a steroid 'problem'; namely, he was unable periodically to abstain from steroids in order to allow his body to detoxify. On one occasion this much talked about 20 stone bulk of a man said to me: 'Oh well, at least I can try and be the biggest in the grave yard' (Field Diary, 11 March 1995: Olympia Gym). Such fatalism contrasts with the individualist and hierarchist tendencies of many bodybuilders who emphasise responsibility, self-control and the utilisation of (some) scientific knowledge in managing steroid risks (Adams 1995).

Steroid abusers, like deep sea divers persistently engaging in 'inexcusably' risky behaviours, enable other members to differentiate 'normal' (acceptable) and excessive risk (Hunt 1995: 452). 'Deviant cases', subject to gossip and rumour and frequently ridiculed in their absence, reinforce in the collective conscience the boundaries for (im)proper use thus delimiting what is and is not acceptable (Durkheim 1964). Considering the functional aspects of Grim-Reaper's avowed deviance highlights, by way of contrast, the parameters for correct usage. By openly flouting or ignoring subcultural rules, social controls for reducing drug-related harm become readily apparent (Moore 1993), rather than remaining part of the bodybuilders' taken-for-granted reality.

In embarking upon a 'normative' lengthy '*cycle*', three points were made which are consonant with bodybuilders' ideas on '*receptor sites*'. Namely:

- receptors degenerate during steroid therapy, hence it is necessary to cease use at some point;
- drug (side) effects are mediated by '*genetics*', hence the continuous user must be genetically gifted tipping the risk-to-benefit ratio in favour of the latter; and
- because it is widely accepted there are long-term health problems associated with continuous use, the legitimacy of heavy and prolonged usage is linked to successful high-level competition and the possibility of a professional bodybuilding career.

Considering the first point, Grim-Reaper conceded that '*receptors sites*' need to recover through periodic abstinence. One '*gym doctor*' (Sonny, respondent 17) attempted to advise Reaper that steroids would be more effective, at a lower dosage, if he had an '*off cycle*'. While Reaper accepted Sonny's pronouncements, he was afraid of losing any of his current size – an inevitable occurrence with drug cessation. The immediate prospect of sacrificing some of his bulk, for the mediate goal of enhancing steroid effectiveness and greater future gains, just seemed too awful for this individual to bear. Analytically, such steroid abuse can be considered the product of the 'situated rationality' of risk behaviour where emphasis is placed on the immediate incentives of risk-taking which outweigh the more distant gratification of abstention (Bloor 1995: 90–1).

Second, Grim-Reaper's peers claimed he did not have the 'natural' bodily potential to become a successful competition bodybuilder. Both Sonny and Alan referred to Reaper as a 'big bag of water'. An excess of androgens, which convert to oestrogen in male users, simply meant that he suffered oedema. In contrast to more genetically gifted world champions (e.g. John), continual usage did not translate to increased musculature and improved bodily aesthetics. Since Reaper's '*genetics*' meant that he could not utilise the drugs he was taking, the increasingly heavier dosages taken to stimulate a minimal effect simply resulted in an '*over spill*' and side effects.

Third, as a non-competition bodybuilder, there was no objective and clearly defined goal to legitimate Reaper's continuous steroid regimen in his peers' eyes, such as winning a prestigious title and turning professional. Cyclic usage may be a subculturally normalised practice for those who do not compete but continuous usage is not universally accepted. Bodily capital in combination with social capital (prestige, titles, income) render high risk activities reasonable. Reaper's and Meat-Loaf's unimpressive bodybuilding physiques, and the impossibility of them emulating John, simply rendered their continual drug-taking pathological in their peers' eyes.

Experimental investigation: the variability of steroid use

Steroid cycling theory legitimates a highly individualised, innovative and experimental approach to drug-taking. Within a generalised ethnopharmacological framework, participants continually modify and devise seemingly idiosyncratic steroid regimens to suit their own particulars. Similar to 'lay' understandings of risk in the context of HIV/AIDS, abstract and experiential knowledge are both utilised for the purposes of body maintenance (Lupton and Tulloch 1998). This may also feed into vocabularies of motive for variable steroid use. For example, experimenters may justify using different compounds by claiming they wanted to try something different, compare them with other types of steroid and find out what they were like. Weinstein (1980: 583), apparently unaware of steroid ethnopharmacology among bodybuilders, terms this type of justification 'knowledge-ableness' and associates it almost exclusively with drug novices and not the sophisticate.

Although a pre-given ethnopharmacological stock-of-knowledge represents a guide to action, bodybuilders' understandings are clearly drawn from their own accumulated experimentation and experience. This experiential, embodied and personally grounded knowledge is valued because different steroids reportedly exert a variable effect from one individual to the next:

LM: You mentioned experimenting with things. When you first started [taking steroids], do people say to you: 'this might be a good thing to try' and: 'it works for me?'

Steve: Yes, that's right. I've tried things in the past that have done nothing for me. Other people say it's fantastic. I think it is basically what works for you don't [necessarily] work for somebody else.

LM: It is just like changing things [steroids] and adding things?

Steve: Yes. You have just got to, trial and error, and try to get out the things that work for you and stick at it.

(Interview: Respondent 31)

This experimental investigation leads to the identification of various compounds, or a particular '*stack*', exerting a more favourable effect than any number of alternative steroid regimens. However, once an effective course has been devised, tried and tested, experimentation may continue in order to confound drug tolerance:

Soccer: My usual stack of Deca and Stromba works for me, and that's my basic cycle. It's my bread and butter course which I will return to time and again. I used that stack last time though, so it makes sense to go onto something different with this cycle that I'm planning on starting next week. If I didn't [change drugs] then my receptors will just get too used to Deca and Stromba, it won't work as well and I would probably have to up [increase] the dosage which is something I would like to avoid if possible. I'm gonna give Masteron [injectable anabolic] a go for the first time with Pink Stars [oral androgenic]. I'll not take too many Pink Stars because I don't want the old bitch tit to flare up. It'll be interesting to see how I react to it, while giving my body a rest from my usual stack.

(Field Diary, 19 March 1995: Soccer's home)

Clearly, while a course may work perfectly well for a bodybuilder, there are so many possible combinations and variations that there may be a more effective course awaiting discovery:

LM: What's your best combination [of steroids]?

Steve: I've put Deca with Parabolan [injectable androgenic] in the past and I still do.

LM: You're not using those at the moment are you?

Steve: No.

LM: So if that's the best one why have you changed it?

Steve: Because the ones I'm doing now I haven't tried before. The Testoviron [injectable androgenic] I haven't tried that before either. I used Dianabol and that's worked for me so I'll use that anyway. I have just gone on this Primobolan and I have never used that before either so it is just trial and error again.

(Interview: Respondent 31)

For bodybuilders an 'effective' and 'safer' steroid course entails identifying specific compounds and tailoring the dosage to optimise results with a minimum of immediate and perceptible side effects. Bodybuilding ethnopharmacologists, in reflexively monitoring their bodies for signs of improvement and danger, are involved in the experimental investigation of various drugs in order to determine a suitable course. Individualising a '*cycle*' by varying dosages and monitoring (side) effects, may be achieved using a technique termed '*receptor-mapping*'. Duchaine (1989: 48) describes '*receptor-mapping*' as a 'quasi-scientific way of optimally adjusting the dosage of a steroid to an individual'. Phillips (1991: 19–20), after describing how some users keep a record of steroids taken, weight and strength increases, various other effects and side effects, adds that while 'receptor mapping is not a science … for some it has proven to be an invaluable source of personal information'.

Drawing graphs and recording other relevant data may assist the user when self-monitoring dosage dependent steroid (side) effects (Phillips 1991: 19). Some bodybuilders keep systematic records of relevant drug information. For instance, one respondent described the methodical approach of a close friend and former steroid-using bodybuilder. This bodybuilder 'tried all the different ones' and reportedly kept a detailed diary, including information on dose related (side) effects (Interview: Respondent 33). Soccer also informed me that he kept a 'steroid diary'. Most users simply employ commonsense as a form of 'receptor-mapping' (Phillips 1991: 20). For example, if an athlete took 200 milligrams of 'Deca' a week and experienced good strength and weight gains, while noticing no side effects, this dose could be suspected to be optimal. Experimenting with 400 milligrams per week may bring on some side effects but no more gains. In this case, the lower dosage is preferred (Phillips 1991: 20). To a large extent, 'receptor-mapping' with a lower dosage before increasing the amount requires patience if the user is to observe mediate steroid effects. The following statement by a body-builder about his first 'bulking cycle' suggests that such experimentation may also entail flouting 'received wisdom':

Mick: I was using real low [dosages of] steroids. The first twelve weeks was just two Dianabol a day. One mil [100 milligrams per millilitre] of Deca for six weeks and 2 for six weeks. That was one twelve week cycle [...] Everybody was saying: 'it's pointless in taking two [Dianabol a day]'. But I just took two and see what happens.

LM: Did you respond from that?

Mick: Yes, I went up [from 14 stone] to 16 stone, so something must have happened.

(Interview: Respondent 22)

According to this junior bodybuilding champion, his modest 'chemistry experi-ment' was successful: optimal results were obtained with a minimal dosage. Potential health risks were reportedly reduced to a minimum, lending weight to the owner of Olympia Gym's ethnopharmacological slogan 'less is best'.

The social distribution of ethnopharmacological knowledge

Various orientations and degrees of integration into bodybuilding subculture have a bearing upon the social distribution of ethnopharmacological knowledge. This knowledge which, for steroid-using bodybuilders, sets boundaries around uncertainty and is 'good to think with' (Bellaby 1990: 468), is not possessed by everybody regularly training with weights and/or using steroids. This section briefly considers who are most knowledgeable, alongside some speculation concerning why they are more knowledgeable.

Individual goals and projects at hand determine the relevancy of bodybuilding ethnopharmacology. For instance, some participants aspire to build or maintain 'Athletically Muscular/Toned Bodies' (Moderately Muscular and Typically Fairly Lean) as opposed to 'Competition Standard Bodybuilding Physiques' (Sizeably Muscular and Exceptionally Lean). The former subgroup, who have more modest bodybuilding goals, often feel they can develop/maintain their 'perfect body' without chemical assistance. For example, a prisoner, who trained with weights to tone his body and 'keep fit' and who based his understandings of steroids on negative media representations, said:

Ben: I've been tempted [to try steroids]. Yeah. Never taken any though [because] I don't know enough about them and there's too many horror stories. I personally don't know enough about them [...] I've never wanted to go into [bodybuilding] competitions. The only reason I would start taking them if I really wanted to get that big to work towards a goal to enter a competition [...]

LM: So to get an athletic physique, you don't really need to [take steroids], you can do it naturally?

Ben: You can do it naturally. You know you can take the fat off and then build the muscle up and get through the plateau as much as you can get and leave it there. If you want to go further than that, there's only a way that your body can go, and once you want to take it past there, you need something to ... I never wanted to take it past that.

(Interview: Respondent P2)

Other weight trainers, termed 'the fringe' by one experienced bodybuilder (Bill, respondent 24), may be totally ignorant of what steroids actually are. For example, some persons lack the sophistication to discriminate between nutritional supplements and steroids (Goldstein 1990: 77). This was evidenced while interviewing an imprisoned weight trainer who exercised to get 'slightly bigger':

LM: Would you say that anabolic steroids are drugs?

Kevin: Anabolic...What ones are they? Powder drinks and all that you mean?

(Interview: Respondent P9)

The modest 'bodybuilding' goals of these two respondents meant that steroid-taking was not deemed relevant to their projects at hand. Consequently, there was little need for these weight trainers to possess an ethnopharmacological knowledge. Other people who try steroids change their structure of relevances; in so doing, ethnopharmacological knowledge becomes more relevant to their interests at hand.

However, steroid users may not necessarily be knowledgeable about the substances they take. This is especially the case if the user is not integrated into bodybuilding subculture. The bodybuilder quoted below, for instance, described the occasion eight years previously when he first used steroids. This occurred before he had embarked upon a weight-training regimen:

Charlie: The first time I used steroids was years ago […] I had a jab off a friend who had been training for three or four years and I'd seen him go from around 11 stone to around … So that's the first jab I took. In the leg as well – fucking killed. Fucking hell! That's I think down to stupidity like. I didn't even know whether … I could have been injecting into a main artery, like, for all I knew. I didn't know nothing, that was the first time. Eight years ago. That was the first time I ever took any steroid, injected steroid.

LM: You weren't even training then were you?

Charlie: No.

LM: Did you know you had to train as well for the steroids to work?

Charlie: No I didn't have no knowledge whatsoever about training and all that. I thought: bang at it and away you go like.

(Interview: Respondent P1)

Bodybuilders, in contrast to other types of weight trainer, aspire to develop extremely muscular, low-fat, symmetrical bodies through the ongoing application of ethnoscientific knowledge. Bodybuilders, who commit themselves to ascetic regimes involving discipline and self-monitoring, are therefore a subgroup of 'weight trainer' likely to possess a sophisticated ethnopharmacological knowledge extending beyond the vagueness of what Schutz (1964) would term a mere 'recipe knowledge'. For these athletes, the use of bodybuilding drugs to enhance physical appearance becomes increasingly relevant. Heightened motivational relevances (sustained interest) render interpretation topically relevant and a protracted (poly-thetic) process of cognition likely (Bloor 1995: 97–9). Here, a greater premium is placed upon acquiring ethnopharmacological knowledge which is instrumental to the 'physique agenda'.

Competitors and non-competitors alike constitute this category of steroid user, where the goal of achieving bodily perfection unites various strata of the body-building community. The following statements, made by experienced members wary of steroid side effects, highlight the importance attached to researching the subject before engaging in personal experimentation. Interestingly, such 'back-ground work' is paralleled among other body modifiers; for example, the 'permanence' of tattoos often prompts caution, careful planning and research among recipients before acting (Sweetman 1999: 57–9). Moreover, by resisting the popular perception of steroid use as an impulsive and ill-thought-out process, bodybuilders utilise 'risk' as a resource for constructing appropriate identities:

Mick: Before I went on steroids it took me six months to sort out what I wanted to take, to find out about steroids, what it was going to do to my system, what was going to happen to me and I think people who don't do that are very stupid. I think you have to look into it seriously before you go on steroids and it has to be what you want.

(Interview: Respondent 22)

Bill: I have never taken steroids willy nilly. I have never taken it without researching the side effects, the possible side effects.

(Interview: Respondent 24)

Len: And when I went on it, it was a well thought out thing. Believe me […] I read everything on it, nutrition, drugs, and made a choice to go on it.

(Interview: Respondent 23)

Phillips' (1991: 9) comment concerning the relevance of information to athletes engaging 'in the risky business of self-administering anabolic steroids' was noted early in this chapter prior to describing steroid ethnopharmacology. This comment made by an indigenous author is noteworthy because it highlights the importance which 'responsible narrators' place on knowledge in maintaining a 'therapeutic course […] centred on getting maximum benefits while confronting the fewest side effects' (Phillips 1991: 9). According to Phillips (1991), and bodybuilders interviewed for this study, knowledge is requisite in surveying the risk environment. Mick (Respondent 22), and others, estimated that approximately 90 per cent of steroid-using bodybuilders (as opposed to weight trainers) are 'educated' about drug effects. He added that it is only the minority who 'don't read up on what they are taking [and] don't talk to people' who risk injuring their health (Interview: Respondent 22). Whether the validity of this point is accepted or rejected, such talk undoubtedly serves as a resource for constructing social identities where narrators present themselves and many of their peers as competent risk assessors and managers.

If bodybuilding subculture incorporates a sophisticated ethnopharmacological stock-of-knowledge, then one question remains: 'which bodybuilders are most knowledgeable?' In offering some speculation, it is to be anticipated that physique competitors (as opposed to Ms Figure-Fitness competitors) will tend to be the most knowledgeable. The immediate and mediate topical relevance of drug-taking in their sport, and the intrinsic motivational relevance for success, renders this subgroup of bodybuilder likely ethnopharmacological candidates. It is no accident that many of the steroid users quoted in this chapter were competitors or former competitors. These data are concordant with recent claims in the medical literature that 'pharmacologic knowledge [among bodybuilders] increases with level of competition' (Anshel and Russell 1997, cited by Augé and Augé 1999: 241). Of course, many participants, including key respondents such as Soccer, have never entered formal bodybuilding competitions and yet take steroids. Similar to competition bodybuilders, these individuals often appear knowledgeable. Luke, another respondent who had never competed as a bodybuilder, similarly possessed a relatively sophisticated ethnoscientific knowledge.

Systems of relevances, which refer to the varying ways in which people orient to perceptual stimuli, are the *bones* of a social theory of cognition (Bloor 1995: 98). Hence, I would argue the influential culture of risk approach (although static and insensitive to the possibilities and constraints of specific social situations) is not entirely incompatible with an embodied phenomenological approach to risk. The extent to which steroid use is thematic and thus topically relevant for a body-builder depends, among other things, upon motivational relevances or sets of interest which guide interpretation and action. But these interests, whether voli-tional or constrained, do not occur within a socio-cultural vacuum. In considering the social distribution of ethnopharmacological knowledge what is clearly important is the extent to which the individual is affiliated to bodybuilding subculture and embraces the bodybuilding lifestyle. This includes the decision to train in hard-core bodybuilding gyms, adherence to bodybuilding training and dietary regimes, socialising with bodybuilders and reading bodybuilding literature. As a general rule, it may be formally stated that knowledge of steroid use is proportionately related to the individual's degree of integration into bodybuilding subculture. This point, emerging from a phenomenologically informed study, is compatible with cultural theories which view risk perception and behaviour as stemming from shared ways of interpreting the world (Wight 1999: 736–7).

Conclusion

In 'risk society' (Beck 1992) the body is viewed as continually placed in a position of defending itself from external threats such as pollutants and toxins (Lupton and Tulloch 1998: 20). If steroids are intrinsically hazardous, and are *self administered* for non-medical purposes, then users are culpable of bodily neglect. Certainly, illicit steroid use may be considered a serious problem requiring legislation, scholarly intervention, education and eventual eradication. If steroid-using bodybuilders uncritically accepted this definition of the situation they would have to concur that they were irresponsible risk takers. However, the well intended goal of eliminating this 'problem' is arguably a product of ethnocentric reasoning, the result of arguing from different cultural premises.

An ethnography of steroid use facilitated a detailed analysis of bodybuilders' ethnopharmacological knowledge which has hitherto only been hinted at by drug researchers. A taxonomy of steroids was presented as well as sophisticated steroid cycling theory. Certainly, this knowledge should not be idealised. Cycling theory, in encouraging careful self-regulation of use and in legitimising continuing and progressive self-experimentation may become both a guard against, and spur towards, self-damage. This is probable with extended habitual use where potentially serious effects on the cardiovascular system are only likely to manifest themselves after many years. Ambitious male competition bodybuilders in particular, who often take high dosages of steroids over prolonged periods, recognise and accept possibly serious long-term health problems. However, these bodybuilders, and other bodybuilders adopting a more conservative approach to their drug use, belong to different cultures of risk from the moral majority. Despite possible and/ or actual steroid side effects, bodybuilders supporting the fundamental tenets of their drug subculture claim ethnopharmacological knowledge minimises steroid-related harm and maximises benefits. Immersion in bodybuilding over time and the embodiment of its presuppositions enables participants to rationalise and sustain possible/actual 'risk' behaviours and preserve competent social identities.

Comparable to prop men in gypsum mines or experienced men working on the kilns in pottery factories (Bellaby 1990: 469), bodybuilding ethnopharmacologists value risk-reducing knowledge, skill and expertise acquired on the job. Comparisons may also be drawn with boxers who, because of their immersion in the game, claim they can minimise 'physical corrosion [through] dutiful corporeal care' (Wacquant 1995a: 83). Correspondingly, and perhaps somewhat paradoxically, bodybuilders' abstract/experiential ethnopharmacological knowledge is not incompatible with the common principle that says one must 'take care of oneself' (Foucault 1986: 43). While ambitious competitors may be more inclined to relegate their long-term health to more immediate concerns, bodybuilding cannot be adequately characterised as an anarchistic drug subculture where health is simply abandoned. Regulatory drug knowledges and practices, which are patterned by gender, are linked to self care and sometimes the care of others. Moreover, steroid abusers, similar to deep sea divers gaining reputations as 'unsafe' among their peers, represent negative role models for 'responsible' bodybuilders attempting to understand the boundaries of normal and excessive risk (Hunt 1995).

The next chapter describes the use of steroid accessory drugs among body-builders (especially physique competitors). It underscores the relevance of flexible ethnopharmacological knowledge in managing potentially serious health risks, creating 'perfect bodies' and the construction of self-identity.

Chapter 6

Steroid accessory drugs

Bodybuilders' ethnopharmacological knowledge of many different steroids and the flexible, individualised and experimental nature of much steroid-taking has been described. However, many different physique-enhancing drugs are frequently used by bodybuilders in combination with steroids:

> At the foot of his bed was his 'treasure chest' as he called it, a footlocker holding scores of magical growth enhancers in bottle and vial form. I couldn't believe the sheer variety of pharmaceutical options available to those involved in the pursuit of muscular accretion. A whole new world opened up to me filled with mystical names and properties.
>
> (Fussell 1991: 119)

In describing the many different pharmaceuticals used by bodybuilders, their anticipated and observed (side) effects, theories and methods of usage, three main points must be recognised. First, this chapter is not exhaustive. Exigencies of space, drug heterogeneity, rapid advancements in modern pharmacology and the 'evolution' of subcultural drug use patterns and behaviours account for this partiality. Second, there is not always consensus among pro-steroid bodybuilders about the 'appropriateness' of particular drugs. This chapter documents the disapprobation of certain drugs among bodybuilders alongside possible justifications and excuses sometimes vocalised by users and former users. Third, certain 'supplements' reportedly containing ingredients exerting 'drug-like' effects are also described.

In offering a bodybuilding drug inventory, each generic class of drug is referred to alphabetically. The chemical substance contained in each generic drug is also noted. Occasionally, a generic class of drug such as Diuretics is taken as a cover term for several drugs containing different chemical substances exerting a similar effect. In such instances, each substance is noted underneath its generic label according to its pharmaceutical name. The proprietary names for different generic copies – specific products containing varying amounts of the generic chemical substance – are numerous and no attempt is made to list all of these. However, a partial list of several versions of a generic drug is provided following the name(s) of the chemical substance(s). If known, the most commonly used generic copy (copies) is (are) italicised. This is useful because bodybuilders often refer to a generic chemical substance, or a generic class of drug, according to a drug's specific proprietary name.

For each drug identified, characteristics and (side) effects are described. Ethno-pharmacological theories and methods of usage – representing justifications which serve as 'constructive rationales' or self-fulfilment accounts (Weinstein 1980: 583) – are also documented. For many bodybuilders, 'underground' pharmacopoeia facilitate calculation of possible risks in conjunction with personally grounded knowledge and casual conversations. Steroid handbooks are therefore treated in the following analysis as a resource in research. However, it is recognised that these texts, similar to members' accounts more generally, are artefacts socially constructed for particular effects; namely, to proclaim a position of responsibility and competence in the surveillance of the risk environment.

Clenbuterol

Substance: Clenbuterol Hydrochloride. Generic Copies: Clenbuter, Pharmachim, *Spiropent.*

Clenbuterol, a medically prescribed anti-asthmatic drug, is available in various forms of administration. Bodybuilders usually take it orally, at a dosage of 0.02 milligrams per tablet. Bodybuilding pharmacopoeia suggest men should take five to seven tablets per day whereas women should take approximately four (Grunding and Bachmann 1995: 50). As a non-steroid agent, the drug reportedly has no masculinising side effects rendering it useful for women bodybuilders.

The '*receptor sites*' possessing an affinity for Clenbuterol are claimed to downgrade rapidly; hence, this drug is also cycled (Phillips 1991: 28). A recom-mended method of usage, according to '*gym doctor*' Sonny, entails taking the drug for ten to twelve days, then two days off, two days on, for six to eight weeks.

One possible side effect is insomnia. Bodybuilders therefore usually take Clenbuterol first thing in the morning.

This drug reportedly exhibits two main physique-enhancing effects. First, similar to Thyroid Hormones sometimes taken by bodybuilders, Clenbuterol assists fat metabolism. However, whereas Thyroid medication acts as a metabolic stimulant, Clenbuterol acts by raising the body temperature. This forces the body to mobilise its fat reserves as an energy source thereby fuelling the heat increase. On a reduced calorie diet, Clenbuterol is considered a useful pre-contest 'cutting drug' (Phillips 1991: 28). Although it might be anticipated that bodybuilders concerned about steroid side effects will use Clenbuterol as a steroid alternative, its effects are reportedly magnified if 'stacked' with 'gear' (Grunding and Bachmann 1995: 50). Experimental data may be taken by individual bodybuilders in order to subject generalised ethnopharmacological knowledge to personal verification or falsification:

Rod: Well, I've used it [Clenbuterol] on its own before now and it never really done a lot to me. It used to give me a bit of a glow or whatever. I did lose body-fat slowly but I found then when I was using it, when I was taking the Dianabol and Anavar, I think the Dianabol and Anavar enhanced the effect of it really and it sort of worked on me like a house on fire then ... Well, the thing is for one, anabolic steroids are known to help metabolise and move the fat around the body, so the fact that it was doing that on top of the Clenbuterol to help burn fat, it really worked well.

(Interview: Respondent 18)

Clenbuterol is considered an anti-catabolic drug. This means it inhibits protein (muscle) breakdown. Many users take Clenbuterol in the belief that it will help them maintain strength and muscularity following a steroid 'cycle' or at least diminish the losses which usually accompany the catabolic phase after a steroid course. According to Sonny, Clenbuterol is valuable in this respect especially if combined with a Gonadotrophic Stimulant such as HCG (discussed later):

Sonny: I think it would help. You're still gonna lose some size but I think it would help us maintain a fair bit of it yeah. If you were using Clenbuterol and HCG [...] It might help you keep most of it [the increase in lean body weight achieved with steroids].

(Interview: Respondent 17)

Again, this generalised prescription is something individual users must verify through personal experimentation and a self-reflexive monitoring of bodily experiences. One bodybuilder, who at the time of interviewing was on his first post-steroid course of Clenbuterol, remarked:

Gary: Well, my strength has sort of stayed there so whether that's due to the Clenbuterol and that, you know, it remains to be seen. But I'm still happy with it at the moment because my strength hasn't gone drastically down.

(Interview: Respondent 42)

Possible side effects include restlessness, palpitations, tremor (involuntary trembling of the fingers), headache, increased perspiration, insomnia, muscle spasms, hypertension and nausea (Grunding and Bachmann 1995: 50). Ethno-pharmacologists, in 'denying injury' (Weinstein 1980: 582), claim side effects are of a temporary nature and usually subside after eight to ten days of use. As noted, users usually overcome possible side effects such as insomnia by taking the drug first thing in the morning. Tremors, another commonly reported side effect, are often considered tolerable or even desirable. Indeed, similar to Becker's neophyte to marihuana (1963), Clenbuterol users must learn to perceive drug effects. Here an immediate bodily sensation representing a possible cause for concern may be interpreted positively: the drug is biologically active and will presumably have a more mediate impact upon body-fat reserves and bodily appearance. Parallels with other groups may also be drawn. While bodybuilders using Clenbuterol differ dramatically from breastfeeding mothers in many important respects, there are parallels in the sense that both groups derive reassurance from uncomfortable embodied sensations. Whether the associated benefit is a nourished baby or a carefully cultivated muscular body, physical discomfort is interpreted positively by both groups through social learning processes. However, some Clenbuterol users report worrying side effects:

Mick: Clenbuterol I have used.

LM: So what do you think of that?

Mick: Scary, very scary. It sent my blood pressure through the roof and gave me wicked bad nose bleeds, really bad nose bleeds [...] It's supposed to burn off fat and hold muscle but all it did was raise my blood pressure sky high [...]

LM: So you stopped [taking it]?

Mick: Yes, straight away as soon as I was having side effects.

LM: So how far into it was you before you started getting side effects?

Mick: A week or so. I wasn't sure whether it was that that was giving me nose bleeds [he was taking steroids as well] so I carried on taking them for a

132

week but I went to see the guy who I get the gear off and he told me it was one of the side effects and the other was high blood pressure so I came off it straight away, and I haven't had a nose bleed since.

(Interview: Respondent 22)

Speculation about long-term health problems was also voiced by some interviewees. For instance, one female bodybuilding respondent – who reported using Clenbuterol to help rid her lower-body of cellulite – heard reports that it strips fat from the body's internal organs. Another respondent, following conversations with a power-lifting clinician, stated Clenbuterol is associated with cardiac problems. However, in the context of other risks and dangers, Clenbuterol-related risk is a *relative* concern (similarly, see Rhodes 1997: 213–14 on HIV-related risk). According to bodybuilding ethnopharmacologists, Clenbuterol is a 'mild' bodybuilding drug and relatively 'safe' – at least, when compared to strong '*androgenic gear*' such as Oxymetholone.

Diuretics

Various Substances: 1) Furosemide; Generic Copies: *Lasix*, Furosemide.
2) Tamoxifen Citrate; Generic Copies: *Nolvadex*, *Tamoxifen*.
3) Spironolactone; Generic Copies: Aldactacine, *Aldactone*.

Diuretics are medicines indicated in the treatment of hypertension and oedema. It is the 'water-draining' effect which renders these drugs useful for bodybuilding. Bodybuilders use Diuretics primarily as a pre-contest aid several days before the competitive event. They do this because judging criteria place considerable emphasis upon the '*ripped and shredded look*' meaning maximum muscle definition. Large muscles are important but it is equally vital that there is a clarity to their appearance. Diuretics help rid the body of subcutaneous water (held beneath the skin) which blurs muscle definition, assisting the bodybuilder to 'polish' the physique. In excreting excess water, competitors with a low body-fat percentage are able to achieve the '*ripped to the bone look*' frequently featured in bodybuilding magazines where the athlete appears exceptionally lean, hard and defined.

The list of generic chemical substances noted above differ in terms of their characteristics and (side) effects. In strict medical terms, Furosemide and Spironolactone are classed as Diuretics, whereas Tamoxifen Citrate is an Oestrogen

Antagonist. (The 'female' hormone oestrogen is not welcomed by male and female bodybuilders because of its effects upon body composition and aesthetics.) However, Tamoxifen also exerts a Diuretic like action, which, according to bodybuilding ethnopharmacologists, is particularly pronounced among women. Hence, it warrants attention along with the 'true' Diuretics.

Furosemide or Lasix as it is more commonly known, is the most potent of all Diuretics. It acts by ridding the body of sodium, chloride, potassium and water (Grunding and Bachmann, 1995: 167). Although injectable versions are available, this drug is usually administered orally two days before a competition. Tablets are available at a dosage of 40 milligrams, exert their effect within the hour, and reportedly last for three to four hours. According to Grunding and Bachmann (1995: 168), bodybuilders experiment by taking half or a whole tablet before observing the effects. Depending on the bodybuilder's condition, the procedure may be repeated.

Furosemide is potentially the most dangerous of all the drugs used by bodybuilders since it poses an immediate life-threatening effect. In ridding the body of essential minerals and salts, an imbalance occurs in electrolytes which may lead to severe cramping and possible cardiac arrest. The following 'cautionary tale' about potassium depleting Diuretics (such as Furosemide) was voiced by one of the sport's elite:

> You get guys training four hours a day when preparing for a show, sunbathing to get a tan [dark skin makes muscles appear more defined] and drinking hardly any water. Trying to get rid of the water, to get harder, that little bit harder for the show. If they've not got the time they take Diuretics which, as well as getting rid of the water, rids the body of potassium and magnesium. You get harder, they squeeze out the water, but you get hard all right – as hard as a corpse. [Name deleted] died because of it, then there was [name deleted] who cramped up on stage. He had to be carried off by four men. They have a glass of water, replenish the water with electrolytes and they're OK.
>
> (Field Diary, 3 April 1995: Seminar by professional bodybuilder)

No competition bodybuilders interviewed for this study reported using Furosemide. This is understandable since commonly used pharmacopoeia point to potentially life-threatening side effects. Furthermore, this Diuretic – in depleting the body of potassium – may deplete water reserves from the muscle, making the bodybuilder appear '*flat*'. Muscles, which should look full, become deflated. Consequently, the risk-to-benefit ratio is heavily tipped in favour of the former.

Furosemide (Lasix) is constructed as a 'risk boundary' by competition body-builders, but potassium sparing Diuretics are deemed less injurious. The generic pharmaceutical compound Spironolactone, known among bodybuilders by the more specific proprietary name Aldactone, is often preferred to Lasix. Aldactone – an oral compound available in dosages ranging from 25 to 100 milligrams per tablet – is claimed to work by excreting sodium and water from the body. Sonny explained how he took Aldactone in addition to the ethnopharmacological reasoning governing his choice of Diuretic. Again, the sophistication of this ethno-scientific knowledge could be used to assuage claims that he was compromising his health:

Sonny: I'll take Aldactone the last four days [before a competition].

LM: What's that?

Sonny: It's a tablet which gets rid of any excess sodium that you might have.

LM: Is that a Diuretic then?

Sonny: It acts as a Diuretic but it's different to something like Lasix, and, if you take a normal Diuretic you just lose the water from the body which includes the muscle as well so you go flat [muscles don't look full], but if you take something like Aldactone it only gets rid of excess sodium in the body, right, and it's the sodium in the body that retains water. It's what I'm after, what I'm trying to do is get rid of any excess water that I might have beneath the skin. Right? So by taking the Aldactone it really tightens you up and gets rid of that excess [water], but you got to make sure you're not taking in any sodium [in your diet]. I take potassium [supplementary salt] as well during the last couple of days [of contest preparation] to keep the water in the muscle because you don't want to lose it from there, just want to lose it from the surface. It's getting the balance right.

LM: Sounds like a science.

Sonny: I know.

(Interview: Respondent 17)

Sally, a high level Ms Physique competitor also used Aldactone instead of the more potent and potentially dangerous Furosemide. Below Sally provides additional technical information on the use of this Diuretic along with certain minerals contained in specific supplements. After stating that competitors monitor their diet to keep sodium intake to a minimum (eating food void of salt and drinking distilled water), she discussed the use of supplementary salts and minerals to overcome potential Diuretic related side effects such as cramping:

Sally: If you're using a lot of distilled water [with Aldactone], it flushes the sodium out of your system – salt – which is what makes your skin tighter. If you take Slow K [supplementary salt] it has got potassium in it but it puts a strain on other minerals [...] if you only take one type of mineral it causes like an influx of that but then a drain on other minerals [...] When I first competed, I went to my chemist and explained what I wanted and he said: 'don't have Slow K. What you want is Sand OK'. It's still got potassium, but it's got a certain amount of sodium and a certain amount of magnesium which keeps the mineral balance so it's not all potassium and no sodium and he said: 'you take that'. And I've never had any trouble with cramping although I've used a Diuretic.

LM: Is that common – oh, it is common cramping [name of professional bodybuilder who was carried off stage after reacting badly to Diuretics] could have done with some of that couldn't he?

Sally: Yeah, but what they take is that Furosemide don't they which is very, very strong.

(Interview: Respondent 19)

When using Aldactone, the duration of application and the intervals of intake generally follows a pre-determined pattern:

Sally: If the show is on Saturday, I take the first one on the Wednesday at half past four [in the afternoon], two on the Thursday – one at half past eight in the morning and one at half past four. Two on the Friday, the same, and the sixth one, half past eight on the Saturday. Why I take them at half past four is so when they start to work, you're not up all night weeing [urinating] and you'll probably find that's how most people take them.

(Interview: Respondent 19)

Tamoxifen Citrate or Nolvadex as it is more commonly known, is the final 'Diuretic' discussed here. As noted, Nolvadex is an Oestrogen Antagonist rather than a 'true' Diuretic. This oral drug, which is medically prescribed to women in the treatment of breast cancer, rids the body of the 'female' hormone oestrogen. This has an obvious appeal to male steroid-using bodybuilders who may risk gynaecomastia (Friedl and Yesalis 1989). However, an additional effect associated with Nolvadex is its mild Diuretic action, making the muscles appear more solid. As commented by Alan: 'it keeps your water down to a minimum. It's like a Diuretic. It keeps you looking that much harder' (Interview: Respondent 21). This effect is claimed to be more pronounced for women. Two female bodybuilders maintained that this drug counters the water retention frequently experienced shortly before menstruation:

136

Sally: Yeah, pre-contest I've used it [Nolvadex] because it gets rid of the fluid.

LM: It's used as a Diuretic? Do you think it is any good for that purpose because a lot of men take it to get rid of Bitch Tits [gynaecomastia] don't they?

Sally: What it does see, it gets rid of the oestrogen in the system where obviously it's the oestrogen that causes the Bitch Tits. So, if a woman is taking it not only – I don't know if you know, but women get a lot of fluid retention because of oestrogen levels, especially during the time of the month. So obviously if you take Nolvadex as a competitive bodybuilder it's getting rid of your oestrogen. But that's why you're getting rid of the fluid, but it's not really a Diuretic but it has a Diuretic like action since it's getting rid of the oestrogen that is causing the fluid retention.

(Interview: Respondent 19)

And:

Zara: I'm thinking of going on Nolvadex.

LM: That should just make your body look harder wont it?

Zara: Yes. Peter [former professional bodybuilding judge] has this theory that women bodybuilders will benefit from it. You see, before I'm due on [menstruating] I put 4 to 5 pounds on [in weight], and it's all water. My body doesn't look good then … If I took it my periods should stop which I'm glad about. Being on is a nuisance.

(Field Diary, 19 June 1994: Temple Gym)

At a typical daily dosage of 10 to 30 milligrams, side effects associated with Tamoxifen Citrate are claimed to be rare. However, nausea, vomiting, hot flashes, numbness and blurred vision are possible (Grunding and Bachmann 1995: 199). In noting possible side effects Grunding and Bachmann add that women may experience irregular menstrual cycles which manifest themselves in weaker menstrual bleeding or even complete cessation of periods. Of course, risk perception occurs from a particular place or perspective; the 'problematic nature' of any object may be reinterpreted positively from a different standpoint. Just as the lethal characteristics of electricity and narcotics are not hazards in the executioner's eyes (Fox 1998: 684), Tamoxifen 'side effects' may be considered wholly desirable from the perspective of the female athlete. For Zara, absence of menstrual flow or, rather, the medical 'problem' known as amenorrhoea, was a functional characteristic of Tamoxifen use to be exploited.

Ephedrine and supplements with a 'drug-like' effect

Ephedrine, containing the generic pharmaceutical substance Ephedrine Hydrochloride, is an oral compound blurring the distinction between 'supplement' and 'drug' within bodybuilding subculture. During fieldwork it emerged that two particular products (Ultimate Orange and EPH.25), legally obtained in Britain from health food shops, either contained Ephedrine or substances exerting a similar effect. Thus, while it is possible to identify various Generic Copies of Ephedrine, bodybuilders using this substance often place specific black-market versions of the drug in the same category as licit supplements containing so-called 'natural' ingredients. Hence, the convention of listing the substance(s) and popular generic copies is overlooked here.

Ephedrine and its counterparts deserve attention for two reasons. First, they are used instrumentally by some bodybuilders for physique enhancement. Second, bodybuilders claim products containing Ephedrine are comparable to amphetamines in their psychological and somatic effects, potentially blurring the distinction between 'bodybuilding drugs' and 'profane' substances enjoyed by 'deviant others'. Correspondingly, there is no clear subcultural consensus concerning the use of Ephedrine. Potential ideological implications – specifically, the possible acceptance and internalisation of negative imputations – therefore emerge in a context where bodybuilders qua responsible risk managers endeavour to uphold a clear distinction between two categories of drug and drug user.

Although Ephedrine is sometimes used recreationally by bodybuilders in certain contexts, bodybuilders contacted during this research claimed they primarily used the drug as a bodybuilding tool. It is this commonly espoused reason which is of primary concern here. This type of self-fulfilment account is most likely to be honoured within bodybuilding subculture because background expectancies render this justification 'reasonable' (Weinstein 1980: 587):

According to subcultural pharmacopoeia, Ephedrine offers the athlete three benefits: it helps burn fat, is anti-catabolic and is a '*training booster*' (Grunding and Bachmann 1995: 108). Ephedrine's effect as a training aid is the most common constructive rationale for usage. Considered a mild form of '*legal speed*' by South Wales bodybuilders, Ephedrine is claimed to help users exercise with greater intensity leading to more productive training sessions and improvements in muscularity. For others, the drug simply enables them to complete a training session if already tired: 25 to 50 milligrams of Ephedrine ingested one hour before training reportedly gives the user an energy burst (Grunding and Bachmann 1995: 108). The owner of Olympia Gym kept a bag of this 'supplement' behind the counter, offering members several tablets if they complained of fatigue. This pharmaceutical dispensary service was provided at no extra cost, along with a complementary cup of coffee with the intention of soliciting a synergistic effect. The socially acceptable drug caffeine is similar to Ephedrine in many respects. Both drugs counter feelings of tiredness. Soccer, a night-shift worker who preferred to exercise straight after work, often relied on a caffeine supplement called 'Pro-Plus' to aid his training. This drug, available from pharmacies without prescription, was useful for pepping up the work-out. Without it, fatigue would inevitably have affected his training session. However, during the Summer of 1995 an 'over-the-counter supplement' became available called 'EPH.25'. Pre-packaged and openly shelved next to buckets of protein powder and vitamin tablets at various body-building gyms, this oral compound contained three pharmaceutical substances: Ephedrine, caffeine and aspirin. (The aspirin is believed to thin the blood, allowing the heart to pump oxygen around the body quicker.) Before this product became available bodybuilders sometimes purchased Ephedrine on the black-market, ingesting it prior to training in combination with the other two drugs. The recommended dosage for each drug being 25 milligrams of Ephedrine, 200 milligrams of caffeine and 300 milligrams of aspirin (Grunding and Bachmann 1995: 108). More often, bodybuilders simply took caffeine or Ephedrine separately. However, the athlete now had the option of taking EPH.25 which was formulated in order to capitalise upon the synergistic effects of these drugs when 'stacked'. Although some respondents claimed this is not as potent as amphetamine, its effects are considered similar.

Soccer tried EPH.25 and found it extremely effective. However, because the body quickly develops tolerance to Ephedrine, necessitating ever increasing dosages, use was reserved for occasions when fatigue would have seriously compromised the work-out. This element of self-control, championed among steroid-using bodybuilders (Bloor et al. 1998), often enables Ephedrine users to justify drug consumption. Although Soccer's use of Ephedrine was occasional rather than habitual, he complained the drug diminished his appetite. While this may be useful if dieting, reduced appetite is not so welcomed among most body-builders who spend most of their time attempting to gain muscular weight. Use was therefore reportedly kept to a minimum by Soccer and other bodybuilders whom I encountered. Amphetamines, while perhaps of some instrumental value in bodybuilding, were also commonly eschewed on similar grounds.

Bodybuilders, who had experimented with various products, claimed EPH.25 was simply a tablet version of another commercially available Ephedrine-based supplement/training aid. This product is called Ultimate Orange. The only difference is that 'Orange' is a powdered formula which the user mixes with water.

Field diary extracts clearly illustrate that '*Orange*' is claimed to exert 'drug-like' (side) effects comparable to more profane substances of abuse. Indeed, while '*Orange*' may possess ergogenic properties – rendering it useful for bodybuilding purposes – side effects such as temporary impotence and insomnia may accompany usage. These 'drug-like' qualities render Ephedrine and related products a risk boundary for some narrators who implicitly excuse experimentation through an appeal to contingent factors (Weinstein 1980: 580):

> I was down at Al's gym and Jack [co-gym owner] said: 'give some of this Orange a try'. It's the American version of it [Next nutrition], the strong one. You're only supposed to take something stupid like a thimble full. I just whacked a couple of scoops into a glass and mixed it with water. I downed [drank] it. Fucking horrible. A little later I went to train and I couldn't believe it. Normally after a warm up I can bench press [chest exercise] three plates [total weight of 140 kilograms] for four reps [repetitions] and then I need a touch [some assistance]. Well, after four reps I was still going, repping out, eight, nine, ten. Fucking hell man! That night I was working the doors [security night club work] and I pulled this piece [met a woman]. I took her back for a shagging [sex] and I couldn't get a hard-on [erection]. My head was gone [couldn't concentrate] with the Orange and I couldn't even sleep for two days either.
>
> (Field Diary, 22 May 1995: Bodybuilder at Night Club/Bar)

If Ephedrine-based compounds blur the distinction between 'drugs' and 'supplements' then the use of '*Orange*' could render the distinction between instrumental and expressive drug-taking equally ambiguous. One bodybuilder, familiar with the effects of Ecstasy, remarked:

> The first time I had it [Orange] I was buzzin' [high] for sixteen hours […] I've taken Ecstasy once and the effect was similar to that. After training I go home on the bus and my head's just gone.
>
> (Field Diary, 10 April 1995: Pumping Iron Gym)

The similarities between Ephedrine, Ephedrine-based supplements and what many bodybuilders consider 'proper' drugs such as amphetamine and Ecstasy prompted some steroid-using bodybuilders to condemn usage:

Dan: [Orange] that's got Ephedrine in it […] at the end of the day it's Speed innit Ephedrine? Speed's pumped full of Ephedrine I think. I mean you don't wanna depend on shit like that. You're gonna start banging the door in [losing self-control] aren't you?

(Interview: Respondent 34)

Similarly, consider the following account voiced by Rod who rejected Ephedrine-based supplements on the grounds that he started to develop an addiction to *'Orange'*. As noted by Weinstein (1980: 581), talk about personal drug addiction enables users to totally disclaim responsibility for drug use while also admitting that such behaviour is undesirable:

Rod: I think things like Ephedrine, well, you know, you start with Nubain as well, you start again at the same sort of category as becoming like what I would call a proper drug abuser. And then it's not long before you want to turn onto Speed, and a lot of people then take cocaine and all sorts then [...] To be honest I couldn't really become addicted, I don't think, to steroids but I noticed last year that I started to become addicted to 'Ultimate Orange'.

(Interview: Respondent 18)

The recasting of Ephedrine as a risk boundary is evidenced in various media of communication. For instance, the 'pro-steroid' editor of one 'underground' body-building magazine writes (Hart, undated: 15):

Another fuck up is Ultimate Orange or it's fancy named competitive counterparts. This shit is packed with Ephedrine Hydrochloride – basically a very mild form of SPEED! This is bad enough and totally useless in the bodybuilding world in my opinion. Why? Well OK, you can boost a workout but what you cannot do is: sleep, make love, think straight, drive or basically anything else. You just sit there – shit faced. That's bodybuilding?

Sensitive to the disparaging view that bodybuilders are 'drug freaks', Hart distances Ephedrine from other drugs abused outside of bodybuilding subculture by acknowledging its instrumental capacity: 'Well OK, you can boost a workout'. However, although adding that Ephedrine is a *very mild form* of Speed, the word 'Speed' is written in upper case letters followed by an exclamation mark. This is unsurprising because amphetamines are often grouped along with 'profane' drugs such as LSD, cocaine and heroin. This link with more common substances of abuse has potential ideological implications for bodybuilders who see their drug-taking as part of an ennobling and self-realising project. Are bodybuilders really able to reject the 'drug taker' label if they use amphetamine like compounds and, in the case of Nubain, a drug comparable to heroin?

Social context and the types of people who use particular drugs are perhaps more significant in defining (in)appropriate activity than pharmacology (*cf.* McKeganey and Barnard 1992: 21). Of most importance here is the instrumental capacity of Ephedrine and related products. If used for physique enhancement, and rationalised in terms of the self-discipline required for building a physique, social identities may remain unspoilt. Here Ephedrine may be used in a manner that is appropriate to competent membership; its use may be congruous with an 'all pervading sense of piety [if] restricted to "on the job" circumstances' (Bittner 1965: 79). This is similarly the case with Nubain, a drug comparable to heroin, which will be discussed shortly.

Esiclene

Substance: Formebolone; Generic Copies: *Esiclene*.

There are various Generic Copies of Formebolone available including Hubernol which is administered as a dragee (sugar coated tablet) or sublingually in the form of drops. However, bodybuilders only use injectable Formebolone (Esiclene).

Esiclene is a '*water-based injectable*' steroid, and is '*fast-acting and short-lasting*'. In bodybuilding it is used almost exclusively as a pre-contest aid. Non-competitors have little use for this compound since all physique-enhancing effects dissipate after only four or five days (Grunding and Bachmann 1995: 119). Although Esiclene is a steroid, indigenous taxonomy and nomenclature does not classify it as a type of steroid. As a localised inflammatory agent, Esiclene has a unique ethnopharmacological use and it is therefore differentiated from other commonly used steroids.

As stated by Duchaine: 'as an anabolic steroid it [Esiclene] is useless [nevertheless] as a contest preparation drug it can mean the difference between winning and losing' (1989: 35). Once administered intramuscularly, Esiclene causes inflammation at the injection site causing the muscle to temporarily increase in size. According to one participant, this swelling feels like a bee-sting – a localised sensation which manifests itself even though the compound contains Lidocaine, a mild pain-killer (Grunding and Bachmann 1995: 119). As Phillips observes, Esiclene is most effective if used in smaller muscles like the biceps, calves or rear deltoids (1991: 33).

A former high level competition bodybuilder described his use of Esiclene. He explained reasons for use, timing of administration and his preferred injection site:

142

Sonny: I've taken it myself, Esiclene, which if you think you've got a weak body-part you put it, you have an injection into that muscle, two days or a day and a half before the competition and it makes that muscle bigger for that, for that competition. It just might, if you've got a weak body-part, it'll bring it up so it doesn't look quite so bad [...] I used to put it in my tricep. I put it in my tricep thirty-six hours before I go on stage, each tricep, and it put a good half inch on your arm.

(Interview: Respondent 17)

Health risks are considered negligible. According to Grunding and Bachmann (1995: 119): 'apart from the pain at the point of injection and, in some cases, a somewhat awkward looking muscle, Esiclene has no significant negative effects'. The observation that Esiclene poses no major threat to health, and can add over an inch to a particular muscle does not mean the risk-to-benefit ratio is tipped in favour of the latter for the majority of (non-competition) bodybuilders. This is because Esiclene's physique-altering capacity is transitory. Competitors are the only subgroup of bodybuilder likely to find this drug useful.

Gonadotrophic stimulants

Various Substances: 1) Clomiphene Citrate; Generic Copies: *Clomid*;
2) Cyclofenil; Generic Copies: Fertodur, Rehibin;
3) HCG (Human Chorionic Gonadotrophin); Generic Copies: *HCG*, HCG-Lepori, Pregnyl.

Gonadotrophic stimulants such as HCG, Clomid and Cyclofenil, are used by male steroid users either during or after a '*cycle*'. Since testicular functioning is often suppressed during steroid use, the intention is to either maintain endogenous testosterone production by the gonads during a steroid course or 'kick start' hormonal production at the end. This is considered necessary in order to avoid the '*crash*' (drastic loss of strength and muscle-mass) sometimes experienced by athletes following steroid use. These drugs are considered ineffective in women because they reportedly work by exerting a positive influence on the male hormone system (Grunding and Bachmann 1995: 65).

The water-based injectable HCG is the most well-known and commonly used Gonadotrophic Stimulant. This pharmaceutical supposedly mimics natural Luteinizing Hormone (LH) in men which stimulates the body's own production of androgens. Maintenance of testicular functioning during a lengthy steroid course, and the prevention of testicular atrophy, is one reason for use. However, HCG is more commonly injected at the end of a course so as to achieve the best possible transition to 'natural training'. The following quotation illustrates how body-builders usually take HCG in relation to their steroid course, alongside perceived effects:

> Len: I always take HCG at the end [of my cycle]. Some people don't, but I think they're being stupid. Yeah, take HCG, get your natural testosterone boosting. I always take three [...] I do my cycle, say I do a three month cycle, and then I leave it a week, so I'll have my last jab on a Friday, and generally then not on the Monday but the following Monday I'll take my first HCG, and then that Friday I'll take another HCG, and then the following Wednesday I'll take the last one. After that, well to be honest for the next fortnight I train better than I do on the gear, that's true, and that's your natural testosterone level, but because you've still got the steroids in you as well, 'cause they're still in your system, and you've got your natural testosterone pumping it out, you're a walking testosterone machine. Do you know what I mean? Train like a mad thing.
>
> (Interview: Respondent 23)

With an increased testosterone production, side effects associated with HCG may be similar to those associated with '*androgenic gear*' e.g. acne, gynaecomastia and water retention. However, if used in the manner described above, side effects are reportedly avoided. Continual use of HCG is not recommended. Ethnophar-macologists claim that steroid receptors in the body down-regulate to such an extent that they become insensitive to endogenous hormone, causing testicular dysfunction and, by implication, muscle catabolism:

> Len: I know guys who just take HCG, only one a week [every week], but that's a problem because in the end your bollocks [testes] over-produce [testosterone] and it works the same as the gear. They're over-producing, so they start shutting themselves down, because the receptor sites are full, so they just shut themselves down.
>
> (Interview: Respondent 23)

Oral medicines such as Clomid and Cyclofenil are also used by male steroid-using bodybuilders as Gonadotrophic Stimulants. As mild forms of oestrogen, these compounds work differently than HCG. Subcultural pharmacopoeia, citing sports medicine publications, report that Clomid and Cyclofenil have a similar effect to HCG even though they have a different biological activity (Grunding and Bachmann 1995: 59–64). This knowledge is sophisticated, drawing from the biomedical model where maintenance of endogenous testosterone is considered the result of 'obviating a negative feedback' in the 'hypothalamo-hypophysial testicular axis' (Grunding and Bachmann 1995: 64–5). Restated, drugs such as Cyclofenil reportedly work by enabling the self-regulating biological body – or, rather, specific interrelated parts of the body such as the mid-brain (hypothalamus), pituitary gland (hypothysis), and testes in men – to continue producing testosterone when production may otherwise diminish (Grunding and Bachman 1995: 59, 64–5). The reported positive influence of these drugs on the male hormonal system, with a minimum of side effects, points to their usefulness in bodybuilding. However, HCG remains the most popular Gonadotrophic Stimulant because it is considered the most effective and is relatively inexpensive (Duchaine 1989: 30).

Human growth hormone (HGH)

Substance: Somatropin; Generic Copies: Genotrophin, Humatrope, Saizen.

Synthetic Human Growth Hormone is an injectable compound medically prescribed to children with retarded growth. Although its effectiveness for adults is disputed (Grunding and Bachmann 1995), athletes generally believe this drug has ergogenic properties, promoting muscle growth and fat-loss. Admittedly, there are those who consider HGH unsuitable for bodybuilding, claiming that the drug 'totally distorts the natural symmetry of the body' (Weber 1996: 188). However, HGH's potential as a non-steroid anabolic agent means that it is included in body-building pharmacopoeia. Indeed, as a non-steroid and thus non-androgenic compound, this drug is reportedly used by female bodybuilders in order to develop extreme muscularity while maintaining a 'feminine appearance' (Grunding and Bachmann 1995: 152). Here female bodybuilders' potentially 'risky' body configurations are recouped (at least to some extent) within the larger project of femininity. At a daily cost of up to $150 US dollars (Grunding and Bachmann 1995), HGH is also the most expensive of all bodybuilding drugs. Hence, use is generally confined to financially secure and ambitious competitors.

In focusing upon bodybuilders' complex ethnopharmacological repertoires, HGH is an interesting compound because drug effectiveness is reportedly only secured with the additive intake of steroids and other drugs (Grunding and Bachmann 1995: 150). After describing the biological activity of HGH, and the synergistic role of other compounds, Grunding and Bachmann ask rhetorically: 'are you still wondering why pro bodybuilders are so incredibly massive, but at the same time, totally ripped while you are not?' Citing Phillips (1990), Grunding and Bachmann (1995: 150) write that the sport's elite are able to become '*freaky*' by practising 'polypharmacy [*sic*] at its finest'.

Two research participants (Alan and Lance) reported using HGH. Their variable drug experiences reflect the dispute within subcultural pharmacopoeia where HGH's effectiveness is a moot point. Lance, following unsuccessful experiment-ation with HGH, remarked: 'it was a waste of money' (Interview: Respondent S03). Alan, after acknowledging some users are very disappointed with the drug, said: 'I was overjoyed with the results I got off it' (Interview: Respondent 21). Similar to Grunding and Bachmann (1995), Alan claimed HGH effectiveness is dependent upon the application of 'correct' knowledge: 'I think it's depending on getting the correct information and then following up the correct information really. You have to put yourself out to be able to be successful, it's as simple as that' (Interview: Respondent 21). Such rhetorical appeals are no doubt significant in establishing narrators as 'individualised experts' in the risk society.

There may be no scientific research showing how HGH should be taken for performance enhancement (Grunding and Bachmann 1995: 153), but general parameters guiding successful personal experimentation are identifiable within bodybuilding subculture. After stating that the drug was too expensive for her to use, Sally commented: 'You've got to get up in the middle of the night, and you've gotta take it and you've got to eat within so long of taking it' (Interview: Respondent 19). Alan provided further details, offering both information and a powerful rhetoric of legitimisation:

Alan: As regards the Growth Hormone, it means two injections a day, twelve hours apart. You can't eat within two hours of an injection because of the insulin effect. So, you have to be able to scale yourself up and get your timing and everything right. It's not a thing you can just do willy nilly because of throwing your body out.

LM: So how would you take it?

Alan: I was getting up and I was having an injection at five o'clock in the morning and the second part of my injection at five o'clock in the evening, because then I was training at roughly half past five so I knew I wasn't going to eat until, say around seven, seven thirty. I would have an injection at five in the morning and have my breakfast then at seven o'clock. How many people are going to be prepared to get up at five o'clock in the morning just to have an injection? But you have to do it correctly.

(Interview: Respondent 21)

The additive intake of steroids is generally accepted as a necessary adjunct to HGH. While female ethnopharmacologists concerned about masculinisation limit their use of the '*androgenics*', Alan claimed testosterone derivatives are an important adjunct. Alan went into considerable detail about the technicalities of taking '*androgenic*' and '*anabolic*' steroids while using HGH:

Alan: Growth hormone basically lives on androgens. It has to be fed androgens. So, I mean, you'll be looking at a testosterone base for it. I would say probably a three to one androgen over anabolic to be enough to get the effect.

LM: What do you mean, three to one?

Alan: On a percentage rate. It lives on androgens so I would say you would have to have a shot of testosterone every other day and perhaps one to two shots of anabolic per week. Tablet wise you would take androgen plus anabolic so you would take, say, Dianabol and Anabol or most people use Anapolon or Anadrol. So, if you take one Anapolon it's the equivalent of ten Dianabol, milligram-wise. So you get the high androgen side of it that way.

LM: It can get quite technical then?

Alan: Very technical.

(Interview: Respondent 21)

If the technicalities of timing, diet and steroids are salient considerations for users of HGH, then careful attention must also be paid to drug preparation. The substance Somatropin is available as a dried powder and before injecting it must be mixed with the enclosed solution containing ampoule:

Alan: It comes in a combined phial if you like. You have the powder on the bottom, you have the solution on the top with a rubber seal. You put it into the pen [container for the drug], as you screw the lid on it pushes the rubber seal down and it's got like a little nidge into the side of the phial and as you get down to there, so the solution runs down and drips onto the powder, dissolving the powder until you've got your 1 mil of GH mixed. Then you click the pen, and that's supposed to measure 1 i.u. [International Unit].

(Interview: Respondent 21)

Dosage and duration of application are also relevant. The recommended daily dosage, as stated in subcultural pharmacopoeia (Grunding and Bachmann 1995: 154), is around 8 International Units. Expense means that many athletes will tailor the dosage according to their finances. Alan, for instance, used 4 International Units per day and still reported excellent results. Cycle length tends to be in the

147

region of six weeks though again the main determining factor is money; those who can afford it reportedly use HGH year round (Phillips 1991: 39).

Side effects associated with HGH are debatable (Grunding and Bachmann 1995: 155). Bodybuilders today use synthetic HGH which, in contrast to its naturally derived counterpart, carries no risk of containing deadly viruses such as Creutzfeldt-Jakob's disease (Duchaine 1989: 74–5). According to Bill, synthetic HGH 'has a very high safety rate [whereas] in the old days you might get HIV if it were around because it was taken from cadavers' (Interview: Respondent 24). HGH reportedly has none of the typical side effects associated with steroids but it is theoretically possible for an excessive and prolonged supply of exogenous HGH to cause acromegaly (bone deformation), gigantism (abnormal growth among the pre-pubescent), diabetes, thyroid insufficiency, heart muscle hypertrophy, hypertension and enlargement of the kidneys (Grunding and Bachmann 1995: 155–6). However, and in a typically postmodernist or, rather, highly sceptical and anti-authoritarian vein, ethnopharmacologists rebuff medicine by claiming side effects are statistically rare. In response to 'the authorities [who like to] present extreme cases of athletes suffering from these malfunctions in order to discourage others', Grunding and Bachmann (1995: 156) write defiantly:

> Among the numerous athletes using STH [HGH] comparatively few are seven feet tall Neanderthalers with a protruded lower jaw, deformed skull, claw-like hands, thick lips, and prominent bone plates who walk around in size twenty-five shoes.

Although this represents an 'external' challenge to medicine within late modernity (*cf.* Gabe *et al.* 1994), bodybuilders claim some (ab)users have experienced problems. It is rumoured that certain elite members have experienced acromegaly of the skull and feet. One bodybuilder's Leukaemia has also been linked to HGH (Weber 1996: 188). Because the prolonged and 'excessive' use of HGH is financially beyond the reach of most bodybuilders, possible 'health risks' associated with duration and dosage are often considered irrelevant.

Nubain

Substance: Nalbuphine Hydrochloride.

If some bodybuilders question the use of Ephedrine and HGH, then there is widespread condemnation of Nubain. There are obvious similarities here between bodybuilders' attitudes towards Nubain and feelings about heroin as expressed by young drug injectors in Glasgow (McKeganey 1990), and drug-using hippies in Sunderland (Willis 1977). Although various drugs were spoken of in a way that signalled their acceptance within bodybuilding subculture, Nubain was widely condemned. Just as heroin is considered 'a mug's game' among young working class Glaswegians injecting Temgesic tablets and the contents of Temazepam capsules (McKeganey 1990: 121–3), most bodybuilders who had injected steroids were highly critical of Nubain.

Briefly popular among some bodybuilders in South Wales (McBride *et al.* 1996), Nubain is an opiate-based painkiller administered by injection. In medicine, Nubain is used as an analgesic and pre-medicant before full anaesthesia prior to surgery (Wormley and Clarke 1995: 36). Often compared to heroin in its effects, this drug is potentially addictive and is generally shunned by bodybuilders: a questionnaire study of 176 steroid users in Cardiff reported only three instances of Nubain use (Pates and Barry 1996). Bodybuilders using Nubain are often considered 'junkies' by their peers – a 'deviant subset' of drug user within body-building. They are typically disparaged on the grounds that they are unwilling and unable to embrace what is sacred in bodybuilding: commitment and hard work. For example, one bodybuilder remarked: 'I think people take Nubain 'cause they're unable to push themselves [while training] and take the pain' (Field Diary, 16 December 1994: Temple Gym).

Mick Hart, the 'pro-steroid' editor of a British 'underground bodybuilding magazine', who is scathing of Ephedrine because of its 'drug-like' effects, also condemns Nubain. In his article 'Nubain: All Pain No Gain' (undated), Hart focuses upon what he sees as the 'intervention of hard drugs into our sport'. He writes: '… like heroin, once jabbed you are literally hooked and FUCKED!' (14). Sensitive to the disparaging mainstream view that bodybuilders are irresponsible risk takers, Hart states: 'I think that the loyal and genuine bodybuilders amongst us will have the strength to resist the temptation of these killer training boosters' (15).

Boundaries or limits determining risk behaviour are apparent within body-building subculture. For example, Nubain's questionable role as a bodybuilding drug, its status as a risk boundary, means that it is uncommon to find reference to this compound in subcultural pharmacopoeia. *The 1995/1996 UK Steroid Guide* (Wormley and Clarke 1995), is one of the few steroid handbooks describing this drug. Even so, they write (1995: 36–7):

[we] had a few reservations about including Nubain in this text since some people who are ignorant of its existence might end up getting hold of some and start using it. But after much deliberation [we] reasoned

149

that it is best to have it included so as to ensure that any unsuspecting and unknowing trainees who have it offered will be knowledgeable and sensible enough to turn it down given the information [we offer].

Because some people have taken Nubain for bodybuilding purposes, the following documents vocabularies of motive for use, including justifications in the form of self-fulfilment accounts and excuses aimed at mitigating responsibility (Weinstein 1980: 583). This entails, among other things, describing drug characteristics, (side) effects, theories and methods of use. Importantly, although bodybuilding ethno-pharmacologists highlight the instrumental capacity of Nubain, as a highly addictive compound it is ultimately seen as a 'hard drug' which should be avoided.

Bodybuilding training can be extremely painful. The analgesic properties of Nubain would therefore suggest the drug has some value as a training aid:

> Some smart fellow reckoned that if Nubain acted as an anaesthetic and painkiller it might have a use in training to numb the muscles being trained, making it possible to subject oneself to extreme intensity past the normal amount tolerable. In use this drug works extremely well making gut busting sessions a regular pastime, and as we all know the higher the training intensity sustained, the greater the growth stimulation and resultant muscular growth (all things being equal).
>
> (Wormley and Clarke 1995: 36)

And, as commented by Hart concerning the perceived benefits of Nubain (undated: 14):

> This product was introduced into the sport a few years ago with forward claims that it would give perfect gains in muscularity, a leaner physique and a boost to the training session like never seen before – it did! People reported fantastic training sessions and were very soon coming out of the gyms looking harder and sharper than ever before.

Of those bodybuilders formally interviewed for this study, Sally, Lance (Sally's husband) and Alan reported experimenting with Nubain. None claimed the drug was a useful training aid. Alan said: 'I tried half a mil prior to training and felt physically sick when I trained' (Interview: Respondent 21). Sally, who 'had the tiniest amount' before her work-out remarked: 'I felt like I was going to go to sleep' (Interview: Respondent 19). Lance, who denied responsibility for use by claiming he was prescribed Nubain by his physician to relieve pain caused by an accident, remarked: 'No [it didn't help with my training]. Psychologically it can because er, a lot of people think "oh, you can't feel the pain." You know? But you can feel the pain. It just takes the edge off it' (Interview: Respondent S03).

Although none of these bodybuilders considered Nubain a valuable adjunct to their work-out, Alan claimed the drug nevertheless has some value as a body-building drug 'if used correctly'. In the following account Alan partly justifies his usage by describing accompanying ethnopharmacological and ethnophysiological reasoning. However, although offering a constructive rationale, he said later in the interview that he was now a former user and voiced the subcultural disapprobation of Nubain. In the following account, this successful steroid-using competition bodybuilder therefore engaged in the strategy of 'scapegoating' (Weinstein 1980: 581) by shifting culpability to somebody who 'told' him to use the drug:

Alan: I was told to use it because of its anti-catabolic effect. Because, your body is either in two states. It's either anabolic or catabolic. If it's catabolic, then it's in a state of disrepair. If it's not catabolic, it's anabolic which is in a state of growth. So, obviously, we all want to be in a state of growth. So I was offered the chance of using it and I used it primarily, as I said, as an anti-catabolic drug.

(Interview: Respondent 21)

Another high level competitor, who did not report using Nubain himself, offered a similar self-fulfilment account which could justify rather than excuse use:

There's Nubain [...] It's also used as an anti-catabolic during contest preparation. It's not an anti-catabolic as such but it has an anti-catabolic effect by relaxing you. You know, with stress the body releases cortisone which inhibits the effect of testosterone so you don't build as much muscle. Before competitions you're under a lot of stress so you need to minimise that. Nubain helps to mellow you out. I suppose you could smoke marihuana instead but that holds water in the body.

(Field Diary, 9 November 1995: The street)

Alan, employing a different model of the drug's action, reported injecting Nubain at particular times to capitalise upon its supposed anti-catabolic effect. That is, at times when his ethnoscientific theorising suggested his body was most likely to be in 'a state of disrepair':

Alan: I took 1 mil per day based on two injections, ½ mil per time [...] ½ mil directly after training when your body is in a catabolic state, and then I tried it, the other ½ mil then I had sometime through the night when it's the other time your body becomes catabolic. It [your body] is catabolic after training due to the fact that you've depleted your body of all its glycogen stores and when you keep yourself down to a low body-fat then obviously the only form of energy is going to come from protein so it counteracts that effect. And then the only other time through the twenty-four hour clock when it [your body] becomes catabolic is whilst you're asleep because it's not fed for eight, nine, ten hours so it's likely to become catabolic through the night.

(Interview: Respondent 21)

Nubain may be injected in one of three ways: intramuscularly, subcutaneously and intravenously. Mode of administration reportedly affects drug pharmaco-kinetics i.e. the time taken to exert a biological effect and the period of activity before the body's metabolism renders the compound ineffective. As suggested below, the pharmacokinetics of Nubain's physiological (anti-catabolic) and opiate-derived psychotropic effects ('the high') are dependent upon type of injection procedure:

LM: What's the difference [in terms of effects] between taking it [Nubain intravenously, intramuscularly or subcutaneously?]

Alan: The difference is the length of time or how quick it gets into your system. If you do it intravenous, before you've taken the needle out of your arm, it's hitting you. It's instantaneous. If you do it subcutaneous [as I was] the effect is say, between thirty seconds and a minute and it [the anti-catabolic effect] lasts for possibly four to five hours. If you do it intravenous it's instantaneous and possibly lasts four to five minutes. If you do it intra-muscular, the [anti-catabolic] effect hits you in about forty-five minutes and it lasts for about seven to eight hours but you don't feel the opiate effect of it.

(Interview: Respondent 21)

Users such as Alan, in redrawing risk boundaries, do not consider Nubain intrinsi-cally dangerous; rather, risk of dependency emerges if the drug is injected intra-venously for expressive rather than instrumental purposes:

Alan: People are taking it as a social drug because of the opiate effect of it and this is where it's become a bad drug for them. And this is where it's become addictive in the fact that it gives them a very relaxed, spaced out feeling. So obviously, if you're having yours intramuscular, you'd have to take a much higher dosage to get that effect than if you're doing it intravenous.

(Interview: Respondent 21)

Intravenous injections, similar to groin injections among heroin users (Rhodes 1997: 222), are often viewed as a risk boundary among bodybuilders. Differential injecting practices between bodybuilders and other types of drug user also enable bodybuilders to engage in 'dividing practices' (Foucault 1983: 208) and the denigration of more 'risky' drug-taking activities. For bodybuilders, Nubain and heroin are comparable; however, if bodybuilders injecting Nubain reject intravenous injections they may still consider themselves responsible risk managers. The retention of competent identity, which is a function of the dynamic and expanding nature of 'normal risk' in a subcultural context (Hunt 1995), may persist even if physiological addiction occurs:

LM: Bodybuilders who use drugs don't see themselves as drug users.

Alan: Yeah. That's contradictory to a point. It's hypocritical if you like, the fact that we use drugs – I feel a little bit like a hypocrite when – it's like I could call Nubain – I'd say it's like a street drug, if you like, because it is opiate-based, so I would say it's like a street drug […] like heroin, cocaine, Crack, whatever. But then [even though I developed a mild addiction to Nubain] I don't class myself as a junkie because I'm not doing it intravenous. To me that's dirty – that's street drugs. Even though I'm taking the same drug. So it sounds a little hypocritical if you like. I can say: 'well, you're taking the same drug but you're doing it in a dirty way because you're putting it in a vein'. Yet I'm taking the same drug. So really I'm no better than him – or worse than him really. It's just that I feel when you're messing with veins, it becomes a dirty habit.

(Interview: Respondent 21)

Finally, it should be stressed that physiological addiction is the most significant risk ascribed to Nubain, rendering this drug an unsuitable bodybuilding compound for most participants. The use of 'cautionary tales' (Goffman 1961) among drug-using bodybuilders, which nearly always relate to third parties, serve to define a normative order, distinguishing the proper from improper for all collectivity members (Coffey and Atkinson 1996). Stated differently, stories are recounted and drawn upon by peer groups to explore their own rules about appropriate behaviour (Green 1997a: 475). Although different injecting practices supposedly render Nubain more or less safe, there is a general consensus that all forms and levels of use must be condemned. In the case of self-administering Nubain, one cautionary tale abounds, possibly dissuading potential users. Here the narrator is Alan, though the same story is told elsewhere (see Wormley and Clarke 1995: 37):

Alan: It's crucified a lot of bodybuilders – there's a guy who won the overall British Championship a couple of years back with NABBA. He's never competed since. Had an addiction to Nubain. He won the British Champion-ship possibly weighing about 14½ stone in Class Three [height class] – he was about 5′6″ in height – about 14½ stone, ripped to shreds. He is now maximum 10 stone, can't train, can't do nothing.

(Interview: Respondent 21)

Conclusion

This chapter described bodybuilders' ethnopharmacological knowledge and self-reflexively monitored use of various compounds. Often used in combination with steroids, these heterogeneous drugs reportedly maximise bodybuilding regimens and enhance bodily appearance. However, such usage may also increase the risks of chemical bodybuilding.

In providing a partial inventory, reference was made to specific compounds such as Clenbuterol, Esiclene and Nubain, alongside generic classes of drug such as Gonadotrophic Stimulants (HCG, Clomid and Cyclofenil) and Diuretics (Aldac-tone, Lasix and Nolvadex). This provided a more detailed picture of drug use in bodybuilding, complementing ethnographic materials presented in Chapter 5. Using members' accounts, it was observed that certain drugs (e.g. Ephedrine and Nubain) may be constructed as 'risk boundaries' (Rhodes 1997) signifying limits beyond which pro-steroid bodybuilders should not venture. However, these drugs' potential for physique enhancement warranted their inclusion in a bodybuilding drug inventory.

Defending 'ontological security', and maintaining a coherent narrative of self-identity, can be fraught with difficulties in risk society (Giddens 1991). If risks are self-imposed then the construction and retention of competent identity may be particularly problematic in a larger society where lifestyle, health and personal responsibility are conjoined (Lupton 1997). For those bodybuilders using drugs instrumentally for bodily improvement, one strategy is to contrast themselves with other types of socially stigmatised drug taker. However, this self-serving differentiation is potentially fragile, especially when Ephedrine and Nubain are used. Because these drugs may be compared respectively and unfavourably to amphetamines and heroin, some steroid-using bodybuilders express concern about the perceived intervention of 'hard drugs' into their sport. Sensitive to the impugn-ment of bodybuilding identity, narrators endeavoured to delimit a normative order through their accounts. This distinguished 'proper' from 'improper' behaviour, ideologically supporting bodybuilders who claim they are not irresponsible drug takers.

While various drugs may be the object of subcultural disapprobation, use may nevertheless be justified by individuals observing proprieties and tolerated licenses that are appropriate to the status 'bodybuilder'. Centrally, this means emphasising instrumentality and self-control over sensual hedonism, impulsiveness and other 'junkie' behaviour. Following ethnomethodological writings on rule use, it is the hallmark of every competent collectivity member to invoke organisational schemes of interpretation 'for information, direction, justification, and so on, without incurring the risk of sanction' (Bittner 1965: 77). Here, competent identity may be retained by drug-using bodybuilders complying with 'organisational rules' while finding in the rule the means for doing whatever need be done. However, Nubain injectors, more so than Ephedrine users, risk disparagement from the self and/or others given a high risk of physiological addiction and the risk of embodying the 'junkie' stereotype. These hazards are deemed highly probable if Nubain is injected intravenously. Recognising possible or actual drug addiction through 'cautionary tales' and personal confessions prompted Nubain users such as Alan to verbalise excuses which diminish culpability (Scott and Lyman 1968). Similar to accounts of steroid abuse, talk about 'deviant' drug-taking is functional. Risk discourse delineates (flexible and permeable) boundaries, establishing perceivably normal courses of action. These discourses may then be utilised by bodybuilders to forge subjective social identities and help create subculturally valorised muscular bodies.

The supposed bodybuilding-steroids-violence connection is the topic of the next chapter. The argument that steroid-using bodybuilders pose a risk to public safety and/or the safety of their partners was much publicised at the time of this research, representing an imposed topically relevant concern requiring negotiation in the social construction of 'perfect' bodies and moral identities.

Chapter 7

Bodybuilding, steroids and violence

Steroids and violence have been causally implicated in recent years, becoming the subject of adverse lay, media and scientific discourse. The risks of steroid-taking reportedly extend not only to users but to the general public by increasing the odds of violent and anti-social behaviour (Lubell 1989: 185). Women have also been identified as victims of physical abuse when their male partners use these drugs (Choi and Pope 1994). Steroid-using bodybuilders, in particular, have been constructed as problematic and have been located in the gallery of violent types along with various other historical figures. Similar to the Mods and Rockers, Hell's Angels, and Skinheads, bodybuilders have become new 'folk devils' (Cohen 1980). Ideological supports enabling gym members to question established medical 'truth claims' and engage in the 'risky' practice of chemical muscle-building therefore acquire particular significance.

This chapter systematically explores bodybuilders' subcultural ideas concerning the alleged steroid-violence link. Centrally, it comments on the ways in which participants may legitimise their alternative conceptions. If existing research is equivocal at best, and has generated a great deal of contradictory evidence (Kashkin 1992), then such an approach is worthwhile. Indeed, because virtually no data exist on steroid users' self-perceptions (Riem and Hursey 1995: 251), the following could contribute 'new' understandings to the academic literature.

Data reporting and analysis is preceded by a brief overview of studies claiming to provide scientific support for the 'Roid-Rage phenomenon. This is necessary for two main reasons. First, these biomedical discourses form a back-cloth to the subcultural claim that drug-using bodybuilders are not necessarily 'dangerous individuals' (Foucault 1988). Second, given the tenacity of the biomedical model of the body (Frank 1990) and patriarchal ideology that seeks to naturalise male

156

dominance, *bodybuilders' theorising* 'recognises' the supposed 'natural' effects of the 'male' hormone testosterone while, paradoxically, also constituting a resource for resisting supposedly certain scientific knowledge.

The alleged steroid-violence link

Similar to commonsense understandings of alcohol's effects on human comportment (Macandrew and Edgerton 1970), conventional wisdom maintains that testosterone – and synthetic derivatives of this 'male' hormone, viz. exogenous steroids – physiologically determines mood states and behaviour. A commonly expressed and widely accepted view, concordant with an essentialist definition of masculinity (Connell 1995), is that steroid-induced detrimental changes include hypermasculine displays of aggression and violence. As stated in one bodybuilding magazine (Brainum 1996: 167): 'Generally, men are considered more aggressive than women because of naturally higher levels of testosterone, which further fuels the concept of 'Roid-Rage'.

In claiming 'Roid-Rage is scientific fact, contributors to the academic literature typically adopt a reductionist epistemology (Pope and Katz 1990). They argue steroids cause immediate/slightly delayed (activational) and/or mediate (organisational) mood and behavioural changes-for-the-worse in the form of aggressive violence. The former, more common variant of the theory, attributes negative behaviours to the over-stimulation of central nervous system androgen receptors; a side effect which is believed to be reversible upon drug cessation (Choi *et al.* 1989). The latter theory links steroid-taking to alterations in brain morphology, long-lasting changes in behavioural responsiveness and dysfunctional reasoning which is independent of subsequent hormonal activity (Kashkin 1992: 388). Psychiatric claims that steroids are associated with irritability, disinhibition, impaired judgement and violent crime (Pope and Katz 1990), are analogous with the near unanimous agreement that alcohol is a 'moral' as well as sensorimotor incapacitator (Macandrew and Edgerton 1970).

Because 'Roid-Rage is a popular assumption among scientific investigators (Riem and Hursey 1995: 249–50), these biomedical discourses help create and make more visible 'dangerous individuals' (Foucault 1988). These forms of knowledge, promulgated by the 'psy-sciences', lend credence to popular claims that steroids will cause uncontrollable outbursts of anger, and by implication violence. Unsurprisingly, many of my ethnographic contacts – in normalising steroid use – contested and revised these biomedical 'truths'. Certainly, many accepted steroids *may* increase aggressiveness and propensities to violence among some current and former (ab)users. There was some concession to conventional understandings. However, bodybuilders embracing the concept of the civilised body (Elias 1978), emphasised the importance of rational thought and control over the impulsive hormonal body. Moreover, in providing a long series of qualifications, and in therefore presenting themselves and/or their peers as mature risk assessors and managers, the supposed steroid-violence (as opposed to steroid-aggression) link was considered very tenuous.

Before focusing upon the data, three caveats. First, although bodybuilders contacted for this study were loath to use steroids as an exculpatory discourse, steroid users *may* attribute their conflict-engendered transgressions to the direct consequence of neurochemical actions (Pope and Katz 1990). In the US criminal justice system, for example, the 'steroid defence' has successfully been used as a plea of mitigation (Moss 1988). In the larger society, steroids, similar to alcohol, have become an acceptable excuse in the form of 'appeals to defeasibility' (Scott and Lyman 1968: 48). Second, in the absence of finely spun subcultural norms ordinarily surrounding steroid use, marginal members' (or other subculturally isolated users') knowledge of steroid effects will be derived from the larger society and the mass media (similarly, see Becker, 1967, and Young, 1972). This, in turn, may increase the likelihood of a self-fulfilling prophecy where the belief, rather than the drugs themselves, lead to negative feelings and behaviours (Bjorkqvist *et al.* 1994, Reim and Hursey 1995). Third, while historical civilising processes underscore the significance of increased bodily control, wilful physical violence (independent of steroid use) is a form of masculine bodily deployment which may be licensed or legitimated at particular times and in particular spaces (Morgan 1993: 77). Respondents constructing 'appropriate' identities in an ethnographic interview may disavow 'uncontrollable' violence but deliberately exercise force in situations where it is hidden, accepted and/or required.

Steroids *per se* do not cause violence: an ethnoscientific theory

Various different and overlapping claims are made by respondents when challenging the supposed bodybuilding-steroids-violence connection. While these 'ethnoscientific' pronouncements perform the same function – they protect the fundamental tenets of bodybuilding as a drug subculture and bolster individual subjectivity – specific claims are considered separately. For instance, the subcultural argument that a steroid user must be predisposed to violence is different from the claim that steroids are only problematic when abused, or the statement that steroids promote aggression as opposed to violence. Of course, steroid users have a range of views on the steroid-violence link, but the views of many experienced bodybuilders and steroid users interviewed for this study clustered in the way reported below. Consequently the objection that steroid-using bodybuilders necessarily pose a risk to public safety carried little weight within this subcultural setting.

Aggression and violence are not synonymous: 'I wouldn't be violent, just snappy'

Reports focusing upon the 'Roid-Rage phenomenon have implied that 'aggression' and 'violence' are synonymous (Goldstein and Lee 1994: 3). However, conflating aggression and violence belies bodybuilders' understandings of mood and behavioural changes. This is evidenced by research conducted among bodybuilders and gym users in the USA (Goldstein and Lee 1994), as well as bodybuilders contacted for this study. Indeed, most bodybuilders implicitly or explicitly differentiated increased aggression from violent behaviour thereby greatly complicating the analysis of steroid/violence relationships (Goldstein and Lee 1994: 5).

This differentiation between aggression (a negative/positive frame of mind, gestures, non-injurious actions, or verbal expressions) and violence (actions intended to cause physical harm) is ideologically important. This distinction allows bodybuilders to concede that some types of steroid *may* enhance 'masculine traits' such as aggression while claiming violence is avoidable if users exercise self-control. In effect, steroid use is legitimated through techniques of neutralisation consisting of a denial of injury (Sykes and Matza 1957). Certainly, there are experienced steroid-using bodybuilders who maintain that these drugs do not exert any mood and behavioural effects whatsoever. However, if a distinction is drawn between aggression and violence, bodybuilders *may* acknowledge that *some* steroids have the *potential* to *exacerbate and/or cause negative feelings in certain contexts* without compromising other people's safety. As indicated below, steroid-related aggression and irritability are also considered activational rather than organisational. Hence, they are largely confined to current use and are reversible upon drug cessation:

Steve: I can get short-tempered. I haven't really got a short-temper but I can get short-tempered while on a cycle.

LM: In what ways?

Steve: Just snappy. I wouldn't be violent. Just snappy.

LM: Just like verbal?

Steve: Very. Less tolerant.

(Interview: Respondent 31)

Len: I can certainly snap quicker [when I take steroids] but I've never done anything about it. Do you know what I mean? I mean my temper rises quicker. I've never hit anybody because of it because I walk away, or I walk out. My temper definitely goes quicker. Definitely. But I'm still in control, still totally in control.

(Interview: Respondent 23)

In stating aggressive feelings may be enhanced during a course of steroids, body-builders differentiate between positive and negative aggression. The former relates, among other things, to feelings of confidence and well-being whereas the latter is a mood state which may be a prerequisite for unwelcome violence. Of course, in feeling more confident users sometimes claim that they are more assertive during day-to-day social encounters (Goldstein and Lee 1994: 6) thus acting in a way that may be interpreted as aggressive (Riem and Hursey 1995: 250). While this may reinforce inequitable gender relations, what is important to the present analysis is the idea that steroid-using bodybuilders do not physically assault people:

Bough: My new girlfriend knows I'm on the gear [...] She's read all these things about it, how it can lead to aggression and make people rape and murder. She said she went to the library and read up on it. I said: 'it's all exaggerated and those people that do rape and are violent are on mega dosages'. I feel more aggressive than normal, but it's controllable. I'm not going to go out and kill somebody. Anyway, it's not that sort of aggression. It's a positive aggression rather than a negative aggression.

Matty: Yeah, it is. The aggression is positive 'cause you feel happy and more confident. You don't go around hitting people.

Bough: I feel more confident, pleased with myself. Because I feel good and in a positive mood I'm less likely to take any shit off anybody.

(Field Diary, 22 February 1995: Temple Gym)

Furthermore, steroid-related aggression may affect the user's sex life: an arena in which masculinity is conventionally acted out. Such aggression was defined positively by male users if it lead to 'increases in their sex drive, longer durations of sexual activity, and more "animalistic" sex' (Goldstein and Lee 1994: 5–6).

Although this may bolster the gendered identity and the self, whether this is actually defined as a steroid-related change-for-the-better is dependent upon the availability of a sexual partner. In the absence of a partner, however, bodybuilders claim steroid induced sexual aggression does not inevitably manifest itself as rape. Additionally, they claim increased sexual aggression is different from actually engaging in violent behaviour which is harmful to their partners (Goldstein and Lee 1994: 6). One steroid user, after attributing his assertiveness to the immediate physiological effects of exogenous male hormones, explained:

Bill: That's another thing that it does, is the sex drive increases.

LM: Does that cause any problems?

Bill: Not really. I mean, a lot of people have used that again in rape cases haven't they? People who use steroids and they've said: 'I've been taking them and therefore it made me more aggressive and more sexual'. It's not sort of like 'I've gotta have sex', or 'I've gotta rape someone'. You know? It's not that sort of thing. I've never found that. It's just that if it was there, you can do it. You know? You know that when – it depends on the partner as well. If you've got an understanding partner or a highly sexed partner then, fine. We're talking about sex four or five times a day for six weeks. One partner I was with and then when I came off it [the steroids] and my sex drive went down, she was like 'hugh!' She kept calling me George from the [British] T.V. programme 'George and Mildred'.

(Interview: Respondent 24)

Increased aggression through steroid use is also positively valued if used instrumentally in the gym (Goldstein and Lee 1994: 6). Indeed, such aggression often enables bodybuilders to lift heavier weights, thus promoting muscle growth. This heightened intensity, which is disciplined, was characterised as 'determination' by some given the negative connotations ordinarily implied by the word 'aggression':

Soccer has been on steroids for about a week now. He claimed he could feel them starting to work on his body. After exercising he asked me if I noticed anything different about his training. I commented that he was training more intensively, and doing more forced repetitions. He said: 'Now am I training more aggressively or intensively? You asked me about aggression in your questionnaire. I'm training more intensively, aren't I? I'm not aggressive in my training … that's where people go wrong. In layman's terms aggression means going around snarling at everyone. I'm not like that. My training isn't more "aggressive", it's more intense'.

(Field Diary, 24 May 1994: Olympia Gym)

The bodybuilder quoted below similarly had reservations about the term 'aggression' since this word is often synonymous with 'violence'. Thus, while he believed steroids may change mood, and this may translate into more intensive training sessions, he said:

Terence: You're not aggressive when you're training are you? I'm an aggressive trainer but the aggression is different. If you understand what I mean? Aggression is well, an example, aggression is: 'I want to rip your fucking head off'. You want to train aggressively, you want to lift the weights but you don't want, nasty, to rip your head off. To me that's aggression [...] It is not violently aggressive then if that's the word I'm looking for?

(Interview: Respondent 14)

Whether this steroid-related feeling is characterised as 'heightened intensity' or 'positive aggression', several bodybuilders stressed that it is directed at weights rather than people. Hence, it is deemed constructive rather than destructive:

LM: You must know a few people who are on the gear [steroids]. Do you notice any change in their attitude? Are they more aggressive?

Bough: Well, I think so, but it's in the gym directed at the weights. Aggression is good like that anyway. You have to be aggressive when you're training to get the results. As I say, though, it's directed at the weights, not to people.

(Field Diary, 2 July 1994: Temple Gym)

Although this form of aggression is considered positive, it is only valued if confined to the gym. If the current user has time off from the gym, some believe 'excess steroid-induced aggression', caused by androgen receptor stimulation, may have no suitable outlet. If this energy is not channelled into the training routine, irritability may ensue:

Debbie: The aggression bit is good, yeah, you know, when you're training. But like on your days off [from the gym] when you've still got your aggression it isn't good. It does put you on a downer and you feel that you're on a downer for no reason. You don't know why you're on a downer but you are. And I find the slightest thing, I snap really, really easy.

(Interview: Respondent 30)

The meaning of aggression is thus context-dependent. If aggression 'spills over' into social relationships causing upset and interpersonal conflict then it is considered negative. It is to be recognised that supraphysiologic doses of steroids administered without exercise do not necessarily increase the occurrence of angry behaviour (Bhasin *et al.* 1996: 6). However, if negative aggression is accepted as a possibility, bodybuilders stress one should learn to control and channel this to positive effect.

To be sure, for some men 'anger is an emotional verification that they are successfully conforming to the dominant masculine stereotype [and] women are especially likely to be victimized by men's anger and violence' (Messner and Sabo 1994: 72). However, it is worth recognising with regards to physical violence and the construction of masculinity that 'power may lie in the manifest control over the expression of anger in physical terms rather than in the straightforward deployment of physical aggression' (Morgan 1993: 76). Some male bodybuilders concerned about 'negative aggression', who were afraid that they would not perceive this and therefore not be able to control it, reportedly relied upon their female partners to point these 'symptoms' out. (Similarly, see Becker, 1963, on learning to perceive the effects of marihuana.) As stated by a competition bodybuilder whose steroid courses could last anywhere up to twelve months:

Alan: I've always said to my wife: 'look, I depend on you telling me if I change, if my attitude changes, if my mood changes. I depend on you to tell me because I won't notice it, so I depend on you. If there's something happening that you don't like, you tell me'. Fortunately, they haven't.

(Interview: Respondent 21)

In sum, according to bodybuilders, steroids *may* exert activational effects which enhance or even cause aggression. However, aggression (a frame of mind, non-injurious acts, gestures, verbal expressions) is differentiated from violence (actions intended to cause physical harm). According to this reasoning, steroids do not inevitably cause socially disruptive behaviour which threatens other people's physical safety. In talking about steroid enhanced 'aggression', bodybuilders were also able to distinguish between positive and negative aggression. The former masculine trait, encompassing feelings of well-being and confidence, is valued among many bodybuilders especially if it leads to an improved sex life and/or more productive training sessions. Some preferred to characterise their attitude in the gym as 'determination' rather than 'positive aggression' thereby eschewing any suggestion that they are abusive or violent towards other people. Negative aggression, which is not considered an inevitable consequence of steroid use, is a context-dependent mood state which – according to responsible narrators – should be controlled. Bodybuilders subject to 'civilising' processes maintain that one may learn to control this immediate/slightly delayed steroid-related detrimental change, and ideally users should monitor themselves during a steroid course thereby avoiding interpersonal conflict. If the user has difficulty in perceiving this activational side effect then they may rely upon an intimate third party to point this out to them.

Distinguishing steroid use from abuse: 'you don't throw a wobbly on a moderate amount'

The following remark made by the owner of Pumping Iron Gym suggests two things. First, there is a relative absence of violence by and among bodybuilders (an observation confirmed during fieldwork). Second, activational steroid detrimental changes are dose dependent:

Rod: I've never, ever, even in the gym itself, known of anybody sort of throwing a wobbly just through sort of using a moderate amount of steroids. Only the one occasion did something happen, but like I say, the boy was abusing it, he was taking way over the amount.

(Interview: Respondent 18)

Most bodybuilders distinguish between use and abuse. Although indiscriminate, unplanned and unsystematic steroid-taking is often equated with abuse, dosage is of primary significance when accounting for potential mood and behavioural detrimental changes. Indeed, total steroid dosage is often considered more important than the duration of the course or the simultaneous use of many steroids, overriding any possible cumulative or interactive effects between various types of steroid and steroid accessory drugs. (However, and as will be discussed shortly, the type of steroid is considered relevant when explicating the supposed steroid-violence link but again negative effects are considered dose dependent rather than interactive.) According to respondents it is to be expected that steroids, like any other medicine, will cause problems if taken in excess:

Soccer: ... there's not been one single case in Britain in the legal courts where it has been proved that steroid use has led to a violent crime. And I say steroid use because there's a difference between that and steroid abuse. There was an interesting programme on T.V. about four weeks ago, *The Cook Report*. It was very sensationalist. They had this woman who had taken the gear, and they said about the various side effects she experienced including aggression. But she said she used one hundred to one thousand times the recommended dosage. Well, a child of six knows that after taking that much there's going to be problems. I mean, do the same with aspirin or even throat lozenges and you're going to get more problems, in fact you'd die wouldn't you? As far as the aggression, you have to distinguish between use and abuse when it comes to such an effect. Just like alcohol, there's people who go out and have a few drinks and they're OK, then there's the total piss-heads.

(Field Diary, 27 June 1994: The Supermarket)

Others endorsed this view. For example, a steroid-using competition bodybuilder remarked: 'I think there is such a thing as 'Roid-Rages but only if you like abuse them, if you take very excessive amounts' (Interview: Respondent 39). His training partner similarly said: 'I think [users who blame their violence on steroids] are lying. Unless they were taking an exceptional high amount then maybe, but other than that I think it is a weak excuse' (Interview: Respondent 44).

As noted in Chapter 5, steroid effects are claimed to vary from one person to the next. Hence, similar to Mullen's (1990) observations on alcohol consumption, use and abuse are relative not absolute concepts. For bodybuilders there is no normative '*cycle*' given different genetic susceptibilities and the belief that everybody is different. Correspondingly it is difficult to state with certainty when steroid use actually becomes abuse.

Rod had his own ideas on this. For this bodybuilder any level of use becomes abuse when it leads to antisocial behaviour. For instance, an athlete could be on a '*heavy course*' and yet avoid trouble; hence, they would be considered a steroid user as opposed to abuser. The following quote is particularly noteworthy because this gym owner, who had countless day-to-day interactions with drug-using bodybuilders, and formed close friendships with many of his clientele, cited mediated violent cases outside his experience which were sensationally reported by the mass media. Here Rod relied on television reports, not personal observations or direct knowledge, when distinguishing between steroid use and abuse:

Rod: I suppose with top competitive bodybuilders they've got to use the gear heavily. [Name of famous bodybuilder] must have used loads but could you say he abused it? He never went off the rails or anything so I'd say that was use. Then you get those guys in the [Welsh] Valleys who knock it back, take everything and are there demanding sex off the wife seven times a day and she doesn't want it. There was a documentary about it. If she says 'no', just pin her down or knock her about a bit then go and pick a car up and try and turn it over. When it gets to that then you've got to call it [steroid] abuse.

(Field Diary, 26 July 1994: Pumping Iron Gym)

While activational detrimental steroid changes *may* be dose dependent, where abuse is a sometime corollary of high level exogenous sex hormones, this is not inevitable. A high dosage might constitute steroid abuse because it leads to socially problematic behaviour, but then again it might not. There is variability in steroid effects just as there is variability in drunken comportment (Macandrew and Edgerton 1970). One steroid injector stressed: 'I have taken them for quite a while, different dosages and I know a lot of other people who have taken different dosages and I have never seen one iota of violence in anybody caused by steroids' (Interview extract: Respondent 36).

Finally, consider the following exchange with a steroid-using junior competition bodybuilding champion. A weight trainer reportedly told him that he became violent towards his female partner while using an extremely small steroid dosage. Bodybuilders' background expectancies concerning the potential psychiatric and behavioural effects of steroids, alongside the subcultural disavowal of violence, rendered this weight trainer's comments unreasonable. However, if this account is valid, one could surmise that the weight trainer felt justified in his beliefs given the publicised view that steroids per se cause violence. In the absence of finely spun subcultural norms ordinarily surrounding steroid use, some individuals lacking a working ethnopharmacological knowledge will be susceptible to negative psychological states and may act upon these (see Young 1972: 40):

LM: Do you think steroids have made anyone you know aggressive or violent?

Colin: No. There was this one, well, he's the same age as me [eighteen]. I don't really know him but this is a classic example. I was chatting to him in town and he started going on about training. And I went: 'oh, you train do you?' And he said: 'oh yeah'. He goes: 'I was on a bit of the gear'. He was saying: 'like I was on two Dianabol tablets a day and I started beating up my girlfriend, so I thought I'd better come off'. And I thought: 'shut up!' I mean, you know? 'Get out of my face!' [...] If you're into the sport like, because most people like bodybuilders, they know what it is all about and, I mean most of them have got wives and kids, I mean they're hardly going to do anything to make them lose their families. So, it's more like the people who've just started weight-training who like to think they're being made aggressive by taking such low amounts that's not even going to affect their body let alone make them aggressive.

LM: It's like two Dianabol. It's probably just the same as...

Colin: An aspirin's going to make you more aggressive than that!

(Interview: Respondent 39)

In summary, bodybuilders claim steroid-related behavioural detrimental changes are unusual but if they do occur then they may be attributed to current steroid abuse rather than current/past use. Contrary to the conventional interpretation of steroid activational effects, violence is considered possible rather than certain among those taking 'excessive' dosages. Varying genetic susceptibilities, and the associated difficulties of specifying normative '*cycles*', render 'use' and 'abuse' relative *not* absolute concepts in bodybuilding subculture. However, any level of use may be described as abuse if violence ensues. As a qualification, negative mood states and behaviours are claimed to be dependent upon a sufficient dosage; that is, an amount exceeding levels necessary for stimulating muscle growth. Steroid-using bodybuilders claim a daily dosage of 10 milligrams of Dianabol, for example, would not exert any noticeable pharmacological effect on physique let alone mood or behaviour.

Being predisposed to violence: 'you have to be like that in the first place'

The general consensus among bodybuilders is that if one has a propensity toward violence, either apparent or potential, then it might be exacerbated during a course of steroids. Steroids (even if taken in 'excessive' dosages) will not turn a 'reasonable person' into a violent one, and it is believed that most bodybuilders are reasonable people. Violence is largely considered an attribute or inclination that is independent of bodybuilding and steroid use:

> After training I showered. In the changing room I got talking to a gym member. We talked about steroids after I told him about my studies. He said he had used Oxymetholone or Anadrol 50 as it is more often known. I asked him whether he believed this drug had any effect on his mood or whether he became violent. He replied: 'No, it didn't change my mood. I wanted to train more, though. I suppose that's the only difference. I wanted to get in that gym and really train. I think, with regards to violence, you'll only become violent if you're violent anyway. You have to be like that in the first place'.
>
> (Field Diary, 28 September 1994: Pumping Iron Gym)

Similarly, as stated by two other bodybuilders during interviewing:

> Jack: I think the people who really explode and do something like a murder would do it anyway. I mean, that type of person is a bomb waiting to go off

anyway. The steroids might be a fact of lighting your fuse, but something would have set them off anyway.

(Interview: Respondent 10)

Mark: In my point of view, if you're a nutter and you take 'em, you'd just be a nutter worse. If you're a normal average person who takes 'em, you'd just be a little bit snappy. You know? Again you'd be just a normal average person in a little bit of a bad mood. That's all. You wouldn't turn a normal average person into a nutter, a natural born killer. You know they don't actually change people's personalities.

(Interview: Respondent 9)

Violence was only seen as marginally related to steroid use. Trajectories producing violence were generally believed to be unconnected with these drugs:

Jack: I know a guy who don't take any [steroids] and he's hopeless. You know? Someone's only got to nudge him and he's out to fight the world [...] The people I know, probably a few blokes that I know like, half of them train and half don't, and there's no difference in the ones who train and the ones who don't. And there's an amount of people within each group who are punchy [enjoy fighting] anyway. Do you see what I mean? You couldn't say all the bodybuilders are punchy and none of them are punchy.

(Interview: Respondent 10)

The temperament and inclination of the person (ab)using steroids are often deemed relevant when accounting for activational detrimental steroid changes. Although various issues are raised in the following excerpt (e.g. learning to control aggressive feelings, designation of certain acts as instances of 'positive aggression', precipitating factors such as stress rather than steroids per se leading to physically aggressive outbursts, un/acceptable targets for violent attacks) the report is noteworthy since Rod claimed *he would have acted the same without steroids*. The only difference regarding his drug enhanced state was that he had more strength; hence, he could cause more damage:

Rod: See that hole in the wall? It's only a dent now as I've plastered over it but it was a hole before [the walls aren't bricks and mortar but wooden partitions]. I tell you I'm glad it happened in a way 'cause if I'd been at home, getting stressed out with the kids running about ... What happened was that I was working with this bloke laying down some mats in the gym. We just had enough rubber to do the job. I'd measured some of it out, thinking that he'd done it the same, but he hadn't. I went out of the room and started cutting it. Well, he cocked it right up 'cause the measurements were all wrong. That really pissed me off. I came out here [to the reception] and head butted the wall. I surprised myself as my head went straight through it. If that had been somebody's head who I'd hated for years I'd have been well chuffed 'cause it would have knocked them right out.

LM: If you'd been stressed out normally [i.e. when off steroids], would you have head butted the wall?

Rod: Well, I might have punched it, or hit it with my head, but not so that I'd put it through the wall. The positive aggression it [the steroids] gave me, I was amazed ... I was really wound up though anyway as a couple of other things happened. I was getting myself psyched up for training as well, getting in the right frame of mind for a good work-out and then my training partner phoned to say he couldn't make it. There was the business with the mats, people were trying to talk to me when I was busy rushing around doing this and that. That's why I put my head through the wall.

(Field Diary, 15 November 1994: Pumping Iron Gym)

The expectation that current steroid-taking *may* enhance aggression and violence among those already inclined to violence is important. Soccer – who gave primary emphasis to the distinction between use and abuse according to dosage – modified this view following Rod's reported outbursts. In so doing, he also placed considerable importance upon the temperament of the user before embarking upon steroids. The following statement was made by Soccer in response to a question posed by a fitness orientated weight trainer who was curious about trying steroids:

Evo to Soccer: I can lose my temper sometimes. I'm the sort of person who gets easily wound up. Do you think it'll make it worse if I take steroids?

Soccer: Well, that's a difficult one. If you're a nice, laid back, easy going sort of bloke then I don't think you've anything to worry about. I think it does exaggerate aggressiveness though if you're normally a bit like that. It just makes it a bit worse. So if, as you say, you lose your temper easily anyway, and somebody cut you up in your car, whereas before you might curse and drive up his arse, on the gear you might end up chasing after him and try and get him to pull over so you can hit him. [This was said tongue-in-cheek.] I'd say it just depends on what sort of person you are.

(Field Diary, 23 May 1995: Pumping Iron Gym)

Two final points. First, some speculated that an individual's pre-existing characteristics and propensities to violence are so important that even if steroids are taken in extremely high dosages, violence is unlikely among those who are normally mild-mannered:

Dan: But I would like to stress for the people who take the gear, I really do think it's up to the individual how they're gonna react. I don't think you can say: 'he's on gear, he's gonna beat...' I mean, I take gear, I'm the last man who wants a fight. Nowadays, you know, I walk away. If someone says 'you're a sissy', I say: 'I'm a fuckin' sissy. I don't want a scrap with you'. Even if I had eight jabs [injections] a week like some people and a handful of tablets, I still can't see in my eyes I'm gonna jump on someone and rip his fuckin' head off. It's the individual. I honestly believe that.

(Interview: Respondent 34)

Second, it is claimed that some people unconnected with bodybuilding deliberately take steroids because they want to become violent. Such a motive is disparaged by gym members and bodybuilders whose primary reason for taking these drugs is to improve bodily aesthetics:

Don: If you were a nut-cracker I think it would be easy to lose your top on some steroids. Well, I know a few people who take it just to lose their top [...] Fucking idiots around town. Take it so they can just fucking lose it [their temper].

LM: Do they train with weights?

Don: No. Just take it to lose their top. [Expression of disbelief on my face.] I know. Incredible innit?

(Interview: Respondent 48)

In summary, according to experienced bodybuilders, a current course of steroids may exacerbate propensities to violence *if the individual is already inclined to violence*. It is reasoned that steroids per se do not cause a dramatic change in personality and action. For the most part violence is considered an attribute or inclination which is independent of bodybuilding and steroid use. In short, those who are violent on steroids are claimed to possess violent tendencies anyway. According to some of my contacts, there are people unconnected with bodybuilding or weight-training who take steroids simply because they want to be violent. If this claim is valid, then such wilfulness is important; it is paralleled among those who treat alcohol as a socially sanctioned opportunity to take 'Time-Out' (Macandrew and Edgerton 1970). That is, where alcohol is used as a socially accepted vocabulary of motive or excuse for violence ('I never would have done it if I had been sober'). It should be added, however, that bodybuilders whom I contacted rarely attributed their own negative moods or behaviours to current or past steroid use.

170

BODYBUILDING, STEROIDS AND VIOLENCE

Changing the body may change attitude: 'becoming an even bigger nutter'

The following statement was voiced by a bodybuilder in response to adverse media attention. In this instance Mark was primarily referring to individual attitude when stating steroids could make an already mentally unstable person even worse. Thus, his comment relates to the previous argument that steroids may exacerbate pre-existing propensities to violence. However, and as will be noted below, 'becoming a bigger nutter' also relates to changes in the size and strength of the body which may lead to a longer-lasting change in negative attitude rendering violence more attractive (Riem and Hursey 1995: 241):

> I talked to Mark about 'Roid-Rage and what he thought about claims made in the newspapers. He said: 'I think 'Roid-Rage is a load of crap. Put it this way, if you're a nutter to begin with then I suppose you'll become an even bigger nutter. As for turning you into a psycho or something, I don't agree'.
>
> (Field Diary, 25 May 1994: Temple Gym)

Respondents often claimed that changing the body through bodybuilding is associated with a more peaceful and easy going attitude: bodybuilders, it was suggested, do not have to 'prove' themselves through violence. (See Morgan, 1993: 76, who relates a similar point to the civilising process, rationality, power and gender.) Even though violence was not publicly advocated by most respondents, some talked about 'deviant cases' who savour confrontation because of their muscular build. In this respect, steroids were indirectly related to violence. Increased muscularity typically enhances feelings of self-confidence and in some cases arrogance. If exaggerated among those with a pre-existing inclination to violence, these attributes may render the individual socially problematic:

Bill: I think with this 'Roid-Rage you get arseholes who take the gear and who then simply have the artillery to be dangerous. They're arseholes anyway, but the gear gives them artillery. The gear makes you feel positive about yourself, makes you more confident and a bit more assertive, and an arsehole with confidence is, I think, a dangerous thing.
(Field Diary, 10 April 1995: Pumping Iron Gym)

It may be inferred from the above account that 'artillery' means 'powerful muscles', rendering those who are arrogant or those with pre-existing personality problems willing and able to act in a socially disruptive manner. Another respondent commented upon mediate effects of steroids on physique, mood and behaviour:

171

Don: You may get your little wimp, who in one or two years might take a whack of gear or something and put a couple of stone on and they are the ones who have the attitude. The ones that go around town and put it about [i.e. fight].

(Interview: Respondent 48)

The following extract is worth quoting at length. The exchange occurred while training in the presence of Noel's wife who, as a non-participant, tended to place primary emphasis upon physiology when accounting for violent crime among steroid-using bodybuilders. After stating 'all that extra testosterone makes them more likely to attack someone [...] having all that extra male hormone is bound to have an effect on how they [steroid users] act', her husband (a former body-builder turned 'body sculptor') countered her reductionist account:

Noel: No, not necessarily, well ... not in that way. There's supposed to be some sort of link, or at least someone has made that claim, but I'm not convinced. Maybe it has been proved there is a scientific link, I don't know, but I think the aggression and violence talked about isn't due to the actual steroids, rather it is a vanity thing, the male ego or whatever you want to call it. I mean, you get someone who starts training and in a matter of time they're bigger, stronger, whereas before they were smaller. Steroids might have been used at some point. I mean, they are used and they make you bigger. We all know that's what they're supposed to do. You get some guy though, he's changed the way he looks and he thinks: 'yes, any trouble and I'm not gonna take it'. If there's any trouble, a potential fight, he's more likely to get involved. I mean, he's got these big powerful muscles and he'll use them if need be. Now, that's not because steroids make him more violent or aggressive. It's more to do with the body and the size he's got. The size and that makes a person more confident and that leads to some people being more cocky. Not everyone, but for a few there's the vanity of it which makes them more arrogant.

(Field Diary, 25 August 1994: Gym in a back street garage)

Riem and Hursey (1995: 249) make a similar point. They state that aggressive behaviour might increase among steroid users not because steroids affect emotional functioning but because a strong build and masculine appearance might facilitate the learning of physical domination as a strategy for dealing with conflict. Similar to organisational effects, this steroid-related detrimental change may be independent of subsequent hormone activity. However, in contrast to organisational effects, negative consequences are a function of changes in the appearance and strength of the body as opposed to structural changes in brain morphology.

172

For the most part, the types of 'bodybuilder' alluded to by Noel are similar to steroid abusers – they are always third parties. However, some did inform me about their own feelings of invulnerability. For instance, Soccer made the following remark after Rod recounted how he verbally threatened some 'troublesome' youths during a night on the town with his wife. It is worth adding that because bodybuilding is possible without steroids, this feeling could very well be independent of current or past use. Of course, by the same token, a more rapid change in appearance through steroid assisted bodybuilding could result in what one of my respondents termed 'The Superman Syndrome':

Soccer: This might sound stupid, but I sometimes feel very confident – too confident – about how big and strong I am. It is daft when you think about it. In one way it's good to feel like you can handle yourself, that you're not vulnerable. If I was walking down the street on my own and there were five yobs hanging around I wouldn't feel frightened walking past them, or through them. That's a stupid attitude though 'cause you might be bigger than them but if one of them whips out a Stanley knife he's suddenly put on three stone of muscle. Also, no matter how big you are, you've only got two fists and two feet. If five lads started you've got ten fists and ten feet heading your way. It doesn't matter how big you are then …I can understand why Rod felt confident and hard enough to have done what he did but can you imagine if a few of them thought: 'yeah, all right, let's do him in'. Or what if they said to themselves: 'I see him walking around sometimes. I'll get him when he's not expecting it'. Rod should be more careful.

(Field Diary, 28 February 1995: Pumping Iron Gym)

An additional point concerns Soccer's reticence. Changing the body with or without steroids may lead to a change in attitude rendering violence more attractive *but only among those who fail to put things into their 'proper perspective'*. As might be anticipated, these individuals are always third parties, except in a few instances when the currently responsible narrator may admit to falling victim to these feelings of magnificence. Bill, who worked as a night club security doorman in the past, said:

When I worked the door I used to think – a big guy'd come in and you'd think: 'oh shit, I wonder if I could take him out if there's any trouble?' Or: 'am I gonna get this guy out of the club?' You know? 'Could I take him out?' When I'm taking gear, I'm thinking: 'I wonder how many punches it'd take for me to take this guy out?' It was never the doubt that I could take him out. And the last sounds like I'm an aggressive

173

person, but that's just the thought, the fleetings of your mind, the fleeting thoughts. You feel 'what could he do against me?' And you feel bullet proof [...] I should clarify this – this is the early part [when I first started using steroids]. When I said that I didn't have – I was adjusting. You know, the instant arsehole and steroids. This is what I was. I think everyone goes through it maybe for the first or second stack if they're using androgens. And it is after all this that I sort of said, I said: 'this is not you' [...] And then, once I came to terms with it, stop playing these stupid games because, you know, you're not bullet-proof. You're not particularly big – like 15, 16 stone is not big. 5´10´´ is not a big guy. There's guys out there is gonna smash you dead! You know? So I wanted to come to terms with it all and I thought about it and thought it all through logically [...] I've never had any problem with it since because I contained it within myself.

(Interview: Respondent 24)

Finally, contrary to Bill's remark that 'everyone goes through [this] maybe for the first or second stack', 'The Superman Syndrome' is not considered inevitable by all users. The following exchange occurred with a junior competition bodybuilder following his first course of drugs:

LM: What do you think about the idea that steroids make people more aggressive?

Larry: I got as aggressive as a lamb. No, I don't think they have that effect. A lot of it I think is in people's minds, maybe it's an excuse. People could take them and get big quick and then that changes their attitude. Like they think: 'wow, I'm big and hard'. And they get arrogant because of the gains they've suddenly made.

(Field Diary, 27 June 1994: Pumping Iron Gym)

In summary, according to many of my contacts, changing the body through the consumption of bodybuilding technologies (including steroids) is often associated with a change in attitude. In short, feelings of confidence typically accompany a change in physique: bodybuilders know they are physically larger and stronger than most people. *If* this feeling translates into arrogance then it *could* lead to aggression, even violence. Members surmised that this is more likely to occur among those who are of a certain mentality ('nutters'). *Although by no means an inevitable consequence* of developing the physique, rapid bodily changes through steroid-taking *could* lead to what some term 'The Superman Syndrome'. This is characterised by feelings of invulnerability. Responsible narrators claim that this 'syndrome' is *potentially* dangerous; hence, 'sufferers' should place things into their 'proper perspective', recognise that they are not invincible, and then control it. Even *if* some do act upon their feelings of grandiosity by becoming violent, 'The Superman Syndrome' is not considered a direct physiological effect of steroids. Rather, it is a socially mediated effect linked to changes in the strength and appearance of the body. Furthermore, 'problem cases' are always third parties, except in a few instances when bodybuilders state that they foolishly acted like this in the past.

Steroid heterogeneity: 'the head-case material'

Bodybuilding ethnopharmacologists, as described in Chapter 5, distinguish between many different steroids in terms of ingredients, strength, (side) effects, etc. They also differentiate between steroids according to potential activational psychopharmacological effects. Because steroids are heterogeneous, some products are deemed more likely to exert a mood-altering effect than others during usage (Goldstein and Lee 1994: 6). The ascription of hazardous characteristics to steroids – and thus the perceived likelihood of an adverse effect – varies within bodybuilding subculture according to type of steroid:

Tim: I think it's certain steroids that have got certain side effects. Testosterone is strong. I mean that's, you usually find with people who get the aggressive turns that that's what they're on. It makes them more aggressive, because I mean it's a male hormone pumping in them and it's a lot more concentrated [than the anabolics].

(Interview: Respondent 16)

Sid: Sometimes I used to get a bit depressed and I found myself getting a bit niggely [irritable], depending on what ones I used to take. On the testos- terones used to make me a bit niggely and a bit short tempered.

(Interview: Respondent 47)

This class of steroid includes specific products such as Halotestin and Dianabol which are sometimes referred to as '*the head-case material*'. Testosterone Cypionate and Anapolon 50 are also considered *potentially* problematic in terms of enhancing negative feelings and propensities to violence. According to Luke: 'I'm only moody when on Dianabol. The Winstrol I've been taking don't make me like that' (Field Diary, 1 August 1994). Bill remarked: 'If there is such a thing as 'Roid-Rage, Cypionate will give you it' (Interview: Respondent 24).

175

Although bodybuilders claim aggressive violence is correlated with particular types of steroid, negative mood and behavioural effects are not considered inevitable:

> I mentioned Luke's feelings of paranoia when on Dianabol to Zara and Bough. Zara replied: 'I can't understand that. If he got paranoid then he must be like that anyway. We [herself and Bough] never experienced anything like that'.
>
> (Field Diary, 14 September 1994: Temple Gym)

The argument that negative mood states or violence are not inevitable with '*androgenic gear*' was also voiced by other steroid-using bodybuilders. Nevertheless, it should still be recognised that implicit in these statements is the view that specific steroids, rather than steroids per se, are correlated with negative aggression and propensities to violence:

Alan: You get a lot of people say when they go on Halotestin, 'it's head-case material'. But I've never encountered anything like that. Never.

(Interview: Respondent 21)

John: How come I've never had nothing like that [a 'Roid-Rage]? And you know, everybody's, through bodybuilding seems some time or other to have taken the same stuff I've taken. You know, we've all used Sustanon some time or another. We've all used Cyps some time or other. They've all used the strongest. There's Anapolon 50. They've all used that some time or other. But I've used that and I've never gone through nothing like that.

(Interview: Respondent 35)

While steroid psychosis is not considered inevitable, some steroid-using bodybuilders did claim certain compounds exert a negative effect upon their moods. However, and in eschewing suggestions of social irresponsibility, narrators said these more potent drugs do not necessarily cause violence. Rather, they simply enhance pre-existing negative traits or feelings during, but not after, the steroid course. Luke, for example, said: 'Dianabol just accentuates it [aggression]. It just makes everything really … if I'm angry anyway it makes me angrier, if I'm hungry it makes me hungrier, if I'm irritable it makes me more irritable. It just accentuates it' (Interview: Respondent 8).

Bill described his mood states while using Cypionate. Here it is acknowledged that it is perhaps the belief regarding the psychological effects of specific compounds which is most important rather than actual physiological effects (see

Bjorkqvist *et al.* 1994, Riem and Hursey 1995). If users believe specific steroids have negative effects then a self-fulfilling prophecy may occur:

> Bill: I've experienced aggression problems with steroids, particularly with Testosterone Cypionate, which is known for its rawness. You know? And that sort of thing. Again, how much of it was self-driven in prophecy – because everyone tells you when you take steroids you'll be a nasty mother, therefore you are. But I definitely experienced problems taking Cypionates so I tend to keep away from those sort of things. I tend to advise anybody that asks for help to just stay away from those sort of drugs as well.
>
> (Interview: Respondent 24)

The expectation of 'negative aggression' while using particular drugs means that some users plan and modify their steroid courses in order to minimise this possibility. For example, Rod made the following remark about specific types of steroid which he and his training partner were using or thinking of using. His ethnopharmacological knowledge prompted him to speculate that a '*stack*' containing two '*androgenics*' (Dianabol and Cypionate or '*Cyp*') would be far more likely to promote aggressive feelings compared to his current course which consisted of one '*androgenic*' ('*Cyp*') and two '*anabolics*' ('*Deca*' and Stromba):

> Rod: I'm on Deca and Cyp, and also the Stromba tabs again. My training partner [who is on the same cycle] isn't getting as good a hit from it as I am [i.e. making good muscular gains] and is thinking of using Dianabol instead of Stromba. I'm not sure though. I don't think I'll go on the Dianabol. I mean, Cyp is such a raw form of testosterone that I can imagine my head going if I take two androgens together.
>
> (Field Diary, 23 May 1995: Pumping Iron Gym)

In summary, negative mood states and violence are not considered inevitable among bodybuilders self-administering steroids. According to bodybuilders' shared ethnopharmacological framework, if aggression is a sometime corollary of current steroid-taking then this is associated with '*the androgenics*' or '*testosterones*' not '*the anabolics*'. Given their potential negative psychological effects, these more potent compounds are sometimes called '*head-case material*' and are deliberately avoided by some users.

BODYBUILDING, DRUGS AND RISK

Discussion: an ethnoscientific reformulation of the 'roid-rage hypothesis

In resisting the idea that all steroids are intrinsically hazardous, many bodybuilders modify activational and organisational versions of the 'Roid-Rage hypothesis. This undermines the conventional, scientifically substantiated view that past and current steroid-using bodybuilders pose a threat to other people's safety. Using those data presented above, the steroid-violence link may be tentatively reformulated. The link is very weak and applies only to a few a-typical individuals possessing pre-existing psychiatric problems. These 'deviant cases' are claimed to be essentially different from the bodybuilding rank-and-file who present themselves as reasonable and sensible people. Synthesising physiological and social components, the conventional steroid-violence hypothesis may be reformulated in the following terms:

> The molecular structure of particularly *'androgenic'* as opposed to *'anabolic'* steroids resembles the 'male' hormone testosterone. According to the taken-for-granted (sub)cultural stock-of-knowledge, concentrations of testosterone enhance 'masculine traits' such as aggression. Thus, it is expected that a course of *'androgenics' may* cause *'negative aggression'* (as opposed to violence in the form of physically injurious acts) which is reversible upon drug cessation. The likelihood of this *potentially* disruptive activational *mood-state* – which *may* manifest itself verbally or in the form of gestures rather than violence – is heightened if *'androgenic gear'* is taken in excessive dosages i.e. if *abused*. Individual genetic susceptibilities vary, making it impossible to state a priori what dosage constitutes steroid abuse. Nevertheless, it is expected that if excessive dosages are taken by individuals with an *existing propensity or inclination to violence* then violence *may* be exacerbated. This propensity to violence is compounded among *mentally unstable androgenic steroid abusers* who are physically stronger and larger through steroids, lifting weights and diet. Given the physique-altering effects of steroids, these drugs *may* have a *mediate effect on violence* by increasing feelings of power and invulnerability as exemplified by 'The Superman Syndrome'. Possessing powerful muscles also increase an individual's ability to inflict more physical damage. Similar to steroid organisational side effects, this ability to cause harm to others may be long-lasting and independent of subsequent hormone activity. However, this steroid-related detrimental change is indirectly related to changes in the strength and appearance of the physique as opposed to brain morphology.

This ethnoscientific reformulation of the 'Roid-Rage hypothesis could be elaborated upon. In explaining supposed detrimental steroid changes, bodybuilders could cite contextual factors intervening between mood change and aggressively violent acts, e.g. working in potentially dangerous occupations such as the police or night club security work, being faced with a jealous partner following an extramarital sexual relationship, conflict with noisy neighbours or argumentative flatmates. In clarifying the dynamics of the steroid-violence relationship, and identifying intervening variables, bodybuilders often emphasise the significance of stress (e.g. familial, work, pre-contest), the additive effects of alcohol (ethno-pharmacologists warn against the combined use of steroids and alcohol, though invariably some ignore this rule), the combined use of recreational drugs, the physiological effects of a calorie-reduced diet on mood. Although no attempt was made to detail these various additions to the conventional theory, it is worth acknowledging them. Indeed, this highlights bodybuilders' reluctance to use steroids as an excuse for violence. This is perhaps unsurprising given the commonly perceived link between bodybuilding, steroids and violence and the popular construction of bodybuilders as new 'folk devils'.

Conclusion

Violence is crudely and stereotypically masculine, and has been described as a possible strategy adopted by those men in ornamental culture who wish to avoid being feminised before an otherwise potentially girlish mirror (Faludi 1999: 37). According to popular images and stereotypes, steroid 'abusing' bodybuilders (most of whom are male) embody this atavistic model of masculinity. The common perception that bodybuilding and steroids are synonymous, and that bodybuilders are, by implication, drug-crazed and violent, is potentially stigmatising. The disparaging view that all bodybuilders represent a risk to other people's safety itself poses a risk to the moral self-image which many bodybuilders present to others and themselves. Correspondingly, how may steroid use be legitimated by 'responsible' bodybuilders?

Qualitative data suggest the steroid-violence relationship may be more complicated than traditionally understood. Importantly, in response to the objection that steroids cause violence, respondents stated a) current steroid-taking may enhance or cause 'negative aggression' but this does not necessarily constitute a social problem because aggression and violence are not synonymous; b) there is a distinction between steroid use and abuse: if used in 'moderation' activational detrimental steroid changes are unlikely; c) steroids may exacerbate an individual's propensity to aggressive violence if that person is already predisposed to violence; d) changing the body through current/past steroid use and bodybuilding may result in a mediate and longer-lasting change in attitude rendering violence attractive; and e) steroids are a heterogeneous class of drug: if aggressive violence and steroids are causally implicated then this only occurs with the more potent testosterone derivatives. However, in challenging the legitimacy of popular and (some) medical discourse, experienced bodybuilders claim there is nothing inevitable about this association.

Finally, the 'Roid-Rage hypothesis was reformulated using bodybuilders' ethnoscientific knowledge. Implicit in members' accounts is a tentative reformulation of the conventional steroid-violence association. Grounded in data (Glaser and Strauss 1967), a formalised and explicit statement regarding the supposed steroid-violence link was offered. This ethnoscientific theory comprises a pharmacological and social component, and contains many qualifications. The mere existence of these qualifications highlights bodybuilders' general reluctance to use steroids as an exculpatory discourse at a time when they were collectively being reconfigured as 'folk devils' or 'dangerous individuals'. Such theorising contains a strong ideological component. Objections concerning the risks of steroid use, even if supported by scientific studies adopting the 'Roid-Rage perspective, are easily challenged by bodybuilders given their sophisticated shared subcultural understandings.

In conclusion, according to bodybuilders' subcultural stock-of-knowledge, steroids per se do not cause socially disruptive behaviour in the form of aggressive violence. This claim is maintained among male steroid-using bodybuilders even though anger, aggression and violence have been linked to the verification of masculine identity within and outside sport (Messner and Sabo 1994). From the perspective of many bodybuilders it is wrong to infer that current and past steroid use indicate personal and social irresponsibility. In the risk society such reasoning constitutes bodybuilders' taken-for-granted reality, serving to legitimate, normalise and sustain steroid use among male and some female bodybuilders.

Chapter 8

Conclusion: constructing 'appropriate' bodies and identities

If we are all charged with taking personal responsibility for our own health, and an affinity exists between bodybuilding and drug-taking, then bodybuilders face possible physical and social risks. Given the sanctity of health in our culture, voluntarily engaging in risk-inducing behaviour becomes morally reprehensible, rendering bodybuilders radically 'other' for those who have the power to define. The demonisation of bodybuilders is compounded given the commonly perceived link between bodybuilding, steroids and violence. In such a context bodybuilding may aptly be described as a community under threat, or, more disturbingly, a threatening community, where participants risk their own and other people's physical and social well-being.

Although by no means exhaustive, this study attempted to understand and theorise (chemical) bodybuilding as an ongoing practical accomplishment. Appreciating the sustainability of this 'dangerous' and 'polluting' pursuit entailed explicating participants' different, more positive, definitions of bodybuilding activities, muscular bodies and identities. Undoubtedly, subcultural disparagement is possible by those members placing themselves outside the positive moment of bodybuilding (Klein 1993). Following Turner's (1999) sociology of body marks, 'cool loyalties' in the form of psychological distance can be expected. However, as illustrated in previous chapters, the perceived 'irrationality' and pathology of bodybuilding, alongside bodybuilding's presumed role as an atavistic or fatal strategy for tackling personal and/or gender inadequacy, may be thoroughly questioned. Bodybuilders contacted during this research often resisted the vocabulary of risk or maintained that self-imposed risks were more or less manageable. The argument that bodybuilding is a self-abusive lifestyle, if accepted by bodybuilders themselves, is related to third parties, formal competitive status and types of dietary and drug regimens. However, self-acknowledged high risk behaviours, especially among experienced competition bodybuilders, may be legitimated in the presence of significant bodily capital.

Elective bodybuilding, a technological way of rewriting the physical body in the flesh (Balsamo 1995: 217), lends itself to many different readings. While disparaging readings abound, the variable project of bodybuilding may be described as a coherent and meaningful lifestyle choice adopted by the denizens of late modernity. For many participants, (non-)competition bodybuilding and instrumental drug use provide a viable identity, a means of anchoring the embodied self. This chapter, sequentially, considers the significance of these ethnographic observations in the social construction of 'appropriate' bodies and identities. An attempt is made to link the sociologies of embodiment and risk, and some possible policy implications for steroid users are identified vis-à-vis tertiary healthcare provision.

Body- and identity-building in risk society

As noted early in this study, according to recent theoretical work the body and the self are less and less extrinsic givens but are instead reflexively constructed and mobilised in the risk oriented world of late modernity (Beck 1992, Giddens 1991). It is argued that within contemporary society, where many people have greater freedom to do what they wish, the body and the self have increasingly become projects to be worked upon amidst continuous warnings about manufactured, globalised and imperceptible danger. However, theoretical arguments on risk and the reflexive construction of the self and body remain at the level of broad claims with little concern for empirical detail (Williams and Bendelow 1998: 104). They do not focus upon the sense-making activities of subjects, the consequences of a reflexive society upon individuals and their subjectivities (Fox 1998: 668).

Preceding empirical chapters indicate that body- and identity-building, at least within this elective technologised pursuit, are conjoined in risk society. In the process of 'becoming other' (Fox 1998: 678), various technologies of the self are used instrumentally by bodybuilders. Powerful synthetic hormones are possibly the most dangerous of these body modification technologies. While bodybuilders could be viewed as 'technophiles' (individualists who see technology as bountiful and liberating), in regulating their usage many could more aptly be described as 'techno-agnostics' or hierarchists who see benefits from new technology only if it remains under their control (Adams 1995: 198). Here drug use is deemed useful even though the beneficial possibilities of science and technology are double edged, creating new parameters of risk (Giddens 1991: 27–8). Bodybuilders' consumption of biochemical resources may be constrained and patterned by (among other things) gendered discourses of steroid (side) effects, the care of the self, finance and the cultural significance of the 'natural' pristine body. That said, 'correct' usage conducted within (flexible) ethnopharmacological parameters is normalised *within* the subculture, even among bodybuilders who abstain from steroids or limit their personal use.

By routinely engaging in behaviours labelled as risk-inducing, reflectivity may be eroded among social actors thereby diminishing the perceived significance of risk (Bloor 1995). However, at a cognitive level risk-taking is potentially damaging to the protective cocoon that defends 'ontological security' (Giddens 1991). Aside from chemical risks, drug-using bodybuilders may be subjected to the accusation that they are locked in a warped logic where muscle accruement is prioritised over self-preservation (Klein 1995). Significantly, many drug-using bodybuilders are able to avoid cognitive dissonance, and preserve a coherent narrative of self-identity, by constructing different understandings grounded in their everyday social reality. In such a context bodybuilders' 'risky' practices represent an opportunity for transformation (Fox 1998: 683–4). Here the term 'risk', rather than denoting 'danger', belongs to the discourse of gambling (Carter 1995). Risk-taking in bodybuilding, similar to risk-taking among others adopting active lifestyles, offers the possibility of gains as well as losses.

Bodybuilders' self-reflexively monitored use of biochemical resources represents a technically sophisticated way of constructing muscular bodies. Physique-enhancing drugs are particularly valued among bodybuilding ethnopharmacologists who successfully construct their bodies within certain parameters: knowledge, dedication, finance and genetics. However, uncertainty concerning *possible long-term drug side effects* (e.g. damage to the liver, kidneys and cardiovascular system) prompts many bodybuilders to adopt a calculative orientation to risk behaviour, or at least to espouse this position in their narratives. Here, perhaps somewhat paradoxically, the possibility of self-other health 'risks' – including steroid induced violence ('Roid-Rage) – may be utilised in the construction of moral social identities.

Bodybuilders contacted for this study appeared to be adept at individualised risk management. Significantly, they used their abilities in this arena as a rhetorical device to present themselves and/or their drug-using peers as technically competent and socially responsible. Recounted instances of steroid abuse by third parties, or the inappropriate use of other substances operating as risk boundaries (e.g. Nubain), facilitated the exploration of subcultural ideas about responsibility, culpability and social identity. Here bodybuilding, drugs and risk fuse in the social construction of 'appropriate' bodies and identities. The doubt and uncertainty which risk-taking (or, more specifically, drug-taking for physique-enhancement) could generate at a cognitive level is reduced. Practical efforts to limit (not eliminate) bodily harm and defend 'ontological security' contribute to the sustainability of chemical body-building, the creation and recreation of 'perfect bodies' within risk society.

Theorising embodiment and risk

> It is not merely that sociologists are becoming aware that the body is 'in fashion', they are increasingly aware that the social actors that populate their theories have bodies that are integral to human existence and thus a central consideration in any theory (Freund 1988, cited by Annandale 1998: 56).

While 'bodies are in, in academia as well as popular culture' (Frank 1990: 131), relatively little social scientific work offers empirically grounded insights into the diverse ways in which specific social worlds are constituted by the embodied agents constituting those worlds (Wacquant 1995a). Most social science publications are 'highly theoretical and interrogate the body separately from its physical, bone, muscle, blood materiality' (Hargreaves 1997: 33). Hopefully the rich data reported and analysed in this book illustrate how qualitative research can contribute to theoretical debate on embodiment and risk.

Recent broad-based theoretical work on reflexive bodies and identities in risk society, as exemplified by Giddens (1991), provides a useful starting point for a grounded study of the body in everyday life. As noted, bodybuilding can be viewed as a lifestyle choice or body-project (Shilling 1993) which has to be reflexively sustained in a context of uncertainty given the erosion of traditional sources of authority and expertise. Through the innovative use of 'risky' technologies of the self, bodybuilding is implicated in processes of individualising the body, the forging of identity and the questioning of medical hegemony. However, in criticising Giddens (1991), Klesse (1999: 20) states that body-projects and the re-ordering of identity '*has not* turned into a free option for all subjects in all situations and contexts [...] the dimension of choice is circumscribed by the complex articulations of gender, ethnicity, ability and class, not to forget location/space'. Reflecting upon preceding empirical chapters, which, in Frank's (1991) words, theorise 'from the body up', current theories of modernity, identity, embodiment *and* risk are revisited.

Gender and class, standard sociological variables of analysis, may pattern involvement in leisure pursuits but they cannot be related straightforwardly to bodybuilding as a 'risky' body-project. The consumption of bodybuilding technologies, similar to contemporary tattooing (Sweetman 1999), is not confined to the male working class. Bodybuilding is currently practised by both men and women from different socio-economic backgrounds (chapter one). And, flexible subcultural prescriptions and conditions for 'success' – the broad-ranging parameters identified in chapter three – are incumbent upon all bodybuilders irrespective of gender. However, while in conditions of high modernity, class, gender and other social divisions are less important, they are not irrelevant. Theorists of modernity agree: 'Indeed, class divisions and other fundamental lines of inequality, such as those connected with gender or ethnicity, can be partly defined in terms of differential access to forms of self-actualisation and empowerment' (Giddens 1991: 6). Correspondingly, there is agreement that body-projects are not free choices for everybody. This is borne out empirically. Bodybuilding is circumscribed by, among other things, gendered ideologies and material resources. These factors are also implicated in risk positions, though not necessarily in the same way identified by Beck (1992).

The affordability of bodybuilding and drug-taking, especially among more committed members, is dependent upon sufficient finances. In that sense, socio-economic position is relevant. While contemporary body modification 'is now popular with an increasingly heterogeneous range of enthusiasts' (Sweetman 1999: 51), material resources are a necessary condition for hard-core bodybuilding. Disposable income is related to risk: the regular and systematic consumption of physique-enhancing drugs (similar to other bodybuilding technologies) can prove expensive. All bodybuilders contacted for this research had some form of regular income, and most were working full-time in the formal economy (chapters one and three). Given the gendered division of labour in British society – women are disproportionately represented in low paid part-time work *and* shoulder heavy domestic responsibilities – structural factors invariably limit women's participation in expensive, time-consuming and potentially dangerous leisure pursuits. Contra Beck (1992: 26), individual wealth and social power may therefore attract risks which are internally rather than externally imposed (Lupton 1997: 89–90).

While gender is relevant, the relationship between bodybuilding and gender is complex. Bodybuilding may be linked (but not straightforwardly) to the construction of masculine identity given its emphasis upon discipline, self-control and the embodiment of force (chapter three). And, at the level of cultural signification 'muscularity' is synonymous with 'masculinity'. While many women may be unable to commit themselves to bodybuilding, many will be unwilling given negative (sub)cultural reactions (Lowe 1998). Hegemonic claims that muscularity and femininity are antithetical constrain women's involvement in bodybuilding. Types of 'athletically muscular' female body may be culturally normative (Bordo 1993), facilitating the growth of Ms Figure-Fitness competitions, but bodybuilding is male dominated. Undoubtedly, the sex/gender system impacts upon body-building practices and resultant muscular bodies. This is the case even though aspects of bodybuilding blur the male-female dichotomy and ongoing bodily development cannot be theorised adequately in terms of antecedent insecurities and the physical embodiment of 'hegemonic masculinity' (chapter four).

In bodybuilding, the articulation of gender circumscribes dimensions of choice and bodily design (Klesse 1999: 20), and these choices are intimately associated with risk (Fox 1998: 679). For example, testosterone use and the cultivation of 'excessive' muscularity among women bodybuilders are constrained by biological and aesthetic arguments (chapter two). Given dominant (sub)cultural discourses about femininity, muscularity and drugs, the social risks of transmogrifying women's bodies become particularly pronounced. Unsurprisingly, there are relatively few female steroid-using physique bodybuilders, and female participants contacted for this research, similar to elite women bodybuilders interviewed by Lowe (1998), invested considerable effort in maintaining their femininity. Phenom-enologically speaking, heterosexual femininity is a volitional ('intrinsic') and, especially among female competition bodybuilders, a constrained ('imposed') topically relevant concern (Bloor 1995: 98). Feminine adornments (hair, makeup), the performance of femininity in bodybuilding competitions (omission of certain poses) and talk about risk (if not actual risk-taking) construct appropriately gendered bodies and identities.

Male bodybuilders, while perhaps not running the risk of losing their mascu-linity, may similarly risk their physical and social selves through drug use and social stigmatisation. In that respect the risks associated with (chemical) body-building traverse gender divisions but gender clearly frames individual risk perceptions, practices and management. Bodybuilding ethnopharmacology, for example, informs differential drug-taking practices between the sexes (chapters five and six). Bodybuilding ethnophysiology, and variable body-projects, are closely implicated in these processes: 'different types of bodily capital determine significantly discrepant probabilities of injury' (Wacquant 1995a: 91).

Dimensions of choice may also be framed by ethnicity. For example, if large sections of the ethnic minority population are materially disadvantaged in an inequitable capitalist and racist society (Nazroo 1997) then bodybuilding (similar to leisure pursuits more generally) may remain a closed option. Conversely, restricted social, economic and political opportunities may channel Black aspirations into the 'physical' areas of sport (Jefferson 1998: 86). Certainly, subcultural ideas concerning Black 'natural' bodily potential are congruent with neo-colonial ideologies of Black sporting excellence (Cashmore 1998: 87). Cultural beliefs about 'innate' biological differences, which, at a societal level, can be seen to reinforce racist assumptions (Sabo and Jansen 1994: 153), may have a differential impact upon risk behaviour among bodybuilders. Some ethnopharmacologists suggest Black bodybuilders should take anabolic steroids rather than the more toxic androgenic compounds (chapter five), or drug use may be discouraged for some time while the athlete gauges their 'genetic potential' (chapter three). Alternatively, representations of the 'genetically gifted' Black athlete may encourage regular and systematic steroid abuse necessary to win high level championships. Again, the relationship between social divisions, body-projects and risk is not straightforward.

In discussing the body as an individual project, Klesse (1999: 20) highlights the importance of other factors which circumscribe choice; namely, ability and space/location. In theorising embodiment, identity and lifestyle choices, these interrelated factors delimiting choice are important alongside time. (Here reference is being made to time as a component of bodybuilding careers, though clearly leisure time is also a socially distributed resource.) At any given point in time different spatially located actors will have different conceptions of bodybuilding depending upon the social distance which exists between them and the subculture. Temporally, the perceptions and knowledge of bodybuilding possessed by an individual will vary during their bodybuilding career. Ethnographic materials are illustrative. For instance, individual ability and willingness significantly to reshape the body is dependent upon knowledge (chapter three). Ethnopharmacological knowledge (chapters five and six), alongside the ethnophysiological capacity to appreciate 'excessive' muscularity (chapter four), are dependent upon social processes of becoming. Ability, or competency, in addition to self-identity, are acquired over time by social bodies through habit and exercise within an embodied habitus (Bourdieu et al. 1991, Shilling and Mellor 1996).

Ability, space/location and time relate not only to embodiment – of doing and being a body in social space (Turner 1996) – but also to risk 'acceptability' and behaviour. This point requires emphasis when evaluating different theoretical approaches to the sociology of risk behaviour. The culture of risk approach (Douglas and Calvez 1990), for example, beside certain empirical inaccuracies in its characterisation of injecting drug users as isolates, is static and fails to account for the movement of individuals from one culture of risk to another (Bloor 1995:

95). Recognising dynamism is significant, however, because health and risk behaviour entail the temporal interplay between individuals, their communities and social environments (Bloor 1995, Rhodes 1997). Such interplay is important in various ways. Variable degrees of attachment to (chemical) bodybuilding may reflect life course transitions (Bellaby 1990) as well as temporally framed stages in the bodybuilding career. Embroilment in bodybuilding, for example, furnishes members with the ability to resist accusations of opprobrium, preserve moral social identities and sustain behaviour under risk. These are important considerations ignored by the influential culture of risk approach (Green 1997a: 476).

Finally, social habituation is significant when theorising the making of bodies in a framework of risk. This phenomenological point, stressing that risk activity may be unconsidered rather than deliberated, runs counter to Giddens' (1991) analytic focus on 'future oriented minds' (Shilling and Mellor 1996). Because risk is processual: '...behaviours that were once seen as risky, or as departures from the norm, may become habitualised as normal over time [they] may be perceived to carry less risk than benefit, particularly if harm is yet to occur' (Rhodes 1997: 220). Self-identified steroid risks, such as oedema, acne and testicular atrophy (all reversible upon drug cessation), are undesirable but often considered *relatively* harmless by users. However, in the absence of medical monitoring, other more potentially harmful effects with long-term consequences (e.g. hypertension, damage to internal bodily organs), may go unnoticed (Korkia and Stimson 1993: 92). Empirically investigating risk and embodiment, while grounding recent theoretical debate about contemporary society, also relates to the practicalities of health interventions (Rhodes 1997) which are considered below.

In bringing this section to a close, it is to be reiterated that there are various theoretical approaches to the study of risk. This diversity is also evidenced in the social study of the body. The topical foci and analytical concerns informing this study underscored the usefulness of an embodied phenomenological perspective. According to McKeganey and Barnard (1992: 51), the attractiveness of phenomenology lies in its ability to explain risk not in terms of deviant motivations but in terms of the context of everyday life. Admittedly, there are contributors to the sociology of risk who consider this perspective too tightly focused (Wight 1999: 739), but phenomenology's concern with the everyday 'world of routine activities' and the previously implicit need not foreclose analysis at a structural or cultural level. As indicated, the culture of risk approach, in attributing variability in risk to differential socialisation in various subcultures, may go some way in explaining different orientations to steroid use. Moreover, for all that is understood that we live in a 'risk society', the sociology of health and illness offers valuable lessons concerning the impact of social structure upon apparently individualised risk exposure (Hart and Flowers 1996: 155). That said, both cultural and broad-based macro-structural types of explanation, abstracted from detailed ethnographic data, can never be fully adequate (Watson 2000: 144). If we accept the ethnomethodological contention that social structures are 'wild' or contingent to emergent factors in specific situations (Robillard 1999), then theorising heterogeneous social phenomena such as bodybuilding, drug-taking and risk necessarily entails a grounded approach (Frank 1991). Phenomenology is particularly suitable for such purposes; it clearly has heuristic value in the empirical study of embodiment and risk. Phenomenology is well rounded, incorporating reference to situations for action, social processes and changing perceptions, calculation and habituation, immediacy and socio-cultural determinants, volition and constraint (Bloor 1995), objective (physical) bodies and animated or experiential (lived) bodies (Turner 1992).

Some policy implications: tertiary healthcare provision

> Drug-related governing policies and authoritative stances are often at odds with the sophistication of the users.
>
> (Augé and Augé 1999: 243)

For egalitarians who view the natural body as fragile, precarious and in danger from human carelessness there is a need constantly to be alert for new technogenic ills (Adams 1995). Drugs, aside from providing some athletes with an 'unfair' sporting advantage, are also widely considered detrimental to physical health. As 'the gremlins of sport' (Todd 1987), steroids and other compounds are (partially) regulated through testing and detection. However, these forms of governance do not extend to the largest segment of the athletic drug-using population (noncompetitive athletes and bodybuilders), and such usage may be considered particularly problematic (Augé and Augé 1999: 218).

This study did not adopt a social problems perspective. As noted by one contributor to the sociology of drug use, such a perspective is aimed at exploring a particular social problem in the expectation of producing information relevant to the control or reduction of the problem at hand (McKeganey 1990: 113). Instead this research bracketed assumptions concerning the pejorative status of bodybuilding and drug-taking for the purposes of understanding the sustainability of these 'deviant' activities. Even so, following growing concern about HIV/AIDS among injecting drug users, sociologists and other social researchers have started to consider the policy implications following on from their work on illicit drug use (McKeganey 1990, McKeganey and Barnard 1992). This is similarly the case among those researching and working with steroid users (Korkia and Stimson 1993, McBride *et al.* 1998).

In noting information which may be of some practical relevance, the following is not governed by an immediate concern to limit the spread of HIV among those injecting steroids. At least in Britain, where needle exchange facilities provide free sterile injecting equipment to steroid users, reports of needle-sharing and the attendant risk of HIV transmission are low (Korkia and Stimson 1993, Lenehan *et al.* 1996, Pates and Barry 1996). This finding is confirmed by this research. Only two interviewees reported giving used injecting equipment to somebody else so they could inject themselves. One of these respondents also reported injecting with used needles given to him; however, he claimed measures were taken to sterilise these needles (boiling in water and soaking in bleach). Significantly, these reported incidents occurred during the 1980s before needle exchange schemes were widely established in Britain. Of course, harm minimisation policies are restricted in the USA: syringe distribution has generated fierce opposition from the 'moral majority' and legal obstacles exist. However, all of my steroid-using contacts reported using sterile equipment and the message about safe injecting practices is widely endorsed by South Wales bodybuilders.

In identifying the practical relevance of this research, particular reference is made here to tertiary healthcare provision. This includes health services provided at sites such as drug agencies rather than General Practitioners' surgeries or hospitals. As noted by Korkia and Stimson (1993: 131–2), existing drug agencies in Britain are well equipped to respond to this new client group; indeed, some have provided separate services for steroid users away from other service agency clientele, viz. amphetamine and opiate injectors. For example, Well Steroid User Clinics (Williamson *et al.* 1993, McBride *et al.* 1998) are important in this respect, performing a valuable harm reduction role in supplying sterile injecting equipment and offering health assessment and feedback. The monitoring of blood pressure, liver and kidney functions is especially welcomed by bodybuilders at these sites and is an empirical illustration of Beck's (1992: 53) claim that risk positions are not determinable by people's own cognitive means, but are instead fundamentally dependent upon external knowledge.

Although of some practical assistance, it should be recognised that drug agency workers may not be credible sources of information to steroid users in general (Korkia and Stimson 1993: 132), and bodybuilding ethnopharmacologists in particular. This, in turn, will limit any efforts made by tertiary healthcare providers when initiating outreach work. This is problematic because a proportion of these users will invariably lack a working ethnopharmacological knowledge but nevertheless consider themselves at minimum risk. Since it is unlikely specialist steroid workers will be paid for by health authorities in Britain, measures could be taken to ensure existing generic drug workers have the knowledge and credibility to work among this population. Hence, one recommendation is that appropriate knowledge, training and credibility is provided to generic drug workers whose knowledge of bodybuilding pharmaceuticals will otherwise be limited. McBride *et al.* (1998: 186) underscore this point by stating drug agency staff, working with steroid users, must be enthusiastic about learning both in and out of the clinic.

As noted, Well Steroid User Clinics perform an important harm reduction role. However, aside from the issue of credibility it should be recognised that these agencies are lacking in other important respects. For example, they do not provide clients with a drug-testing service in order to check drug safety and effectiveness. Nor do they prescribe legitimate pharmaceuticals, the quality of which would be assured. Prescribing steroids, however, is not beyond the realms of possibility (Bhasin *et al.* 1996), and would do much to increase the appeal of service agencies to drug-using bodybuilders. McBride *et al.* (1998), quoting Millar's (1994) attempts at harm minimisation through prescribing steroids, acknowledge this as a real possibility.

In discussing the possibility of drug-testing and/or prescribing physique-enhancing drugs the practicality of these measures should be underscored alongside their rationale. For example, it is acknowledged that an open ended drug-testing programme, where all samples could be subjected to laboratory analyses, will prove too expensive for most users and health authorities alike. A more practicable approach, therefore, would be for samples to be tested at the discretion of staff where there was a case for harm minimisation. Limited funds obtained from the health authority and/or agency clients could then be used to test samples obtained from a new batch of drugs circulating among the local drug-using population. The case for such testing would appear especially strong if clients expressed concern about the quality of a particular batch of drugs. Alternatively, and something which would prove more cost effective than an open ended drug-testing service, would be a programme of prescribing physique-enhancing drugs. This would parallel the efforts of clinicians working with opiate and amphetamine injectors (Fountain *et al.* 1996). While an important rationale for this would be to ensure the quality of drugs – prescribed medicines should be free from contamination – it is recognised that this measure could also prove valuable in controlling dosages. This would be particularly helpful to steroid-abusing bodybuilders who consider themselves psychologically dependent and require assistance in abstaining from drugs or moderating their intake. One problem in Britain is that clinicians may be limited in terms of the range of substances available to them. Certain types of steroids popular among bodybuilders in South Wales, for example, are only produced and prescribed overseas. Hence, there would seem to be a case both for prescribing medicines and testing illicitly procured substances.

Clearly, there is a possibility of ensuring and extending the impact of tertiary healthcare agencies. This could be achieved in several ways. As well as increasing the range of services provided to those attending Well Steroid User Clinics, an interactive role could be established at these sites between sports medicine specialists and experienced drug-using bodybuilders (McBride *et al.* 1998: 187). The goal would be to further knowledge of drug efficacy, paralleling AIDS activists involvement as co-researchers in the design and implementation of drug trials (Epstein 1996). Here visions of 'expertise' would shift, at least to some extent, from the professional to those with indigenous status. This move from 'business suits to grassroots' also parallels trends among health professionals involved with other drug-injecting populations where the emphasis is to work with the community (Rhodes and Stimson 1998).

These suggestions are based upon a recognition 'that the territory of expertise does not always coincide with territory of formal scientific education and certification' (Collins and Pinch 1998: 5). Such a recognition is essential given the credibility gap that has long existed between the medical and athletic communities: the medical profession, contrary to athletes' experientially derived knowledge of drug efficacy, have long claimed steroids are 'fools' gold' (Monaghan 1999b). Even so, there is a cultural congruence between medicine and bodybuilding to the extent that many drug-using bodybuilders would welcome specialist medical assistance. Bodybuilders are generally receptive to health promotion interventions; for example, Korkia and Stimson (1993: 132) note that many steroid users have told their GP about their drug use and some already receive medical monitoring from GPs and others. Undoubtedly, a mutually beneficial role could be established where specialists would be involved in the experimental investigation of physique-enhancing drugs. Trials could be established, similar to that undertaken by Bhasin *et al.* (1996), where (ethno)scientists attempt to devise an array of 'therapeutic' drug regimens aimed at enhancing physique and performance while minimising drug-related harm.

To be sure, science and technology are thoroughly human endeavours and are therefore fallible (Collins and Pinch 1998). And, as is well recognised by bodybuilding ethnopharmacologists, different genetic susceptibilities and changing patterns of drug tolerance will complicate matters. Inevitably, predictions of the long-term health effects of drugs even at low dosages will be an uncertain business: something which is compounded given the long latency period of most carcinogens and toxins and the synergistic effects of substances acting in combination (Adams 1995: 49). Furthermore, in terms of scientists who may possess relevant co-expertise, there are currently relatively few sports medicine specialists, at least in the UK (McBride *et al.* 1998: 187).

Following the recommendations of one indigenous author writing in the USA, a new branch of medicine could be established: 'Physique Augmentation' (Phillips 1997b). Whether, in such a context, medical technology represents a panacea or chimera is open to debate (*cf.* Annandale 1998: 267). Certainly, this suggestion may be criticised; it could be interpreted as an instance of medicine extending its activity and profiting from self-produced risks (Beck 1992: 267). Here medicine aimed at 'correction' (as in surgical augmentation) may be implicated in the social construction of the body as a 'coercive ideal' where 'patients [bodybuilders] pursue with the physician (make that beautician) the cookie-cutter pattern of the recon-structed body' (Fussell 1994: 59). However, for many bodybuilders there are discernible advantages in obtaining medical assistance. The wish to recruit medicine, recently expressed in the bodybuilding literature, has generated a positive response from bodybuilding clinicians (Phillips 1997c: 20). It is proposed that medics – preferably with a personal involvement in bodybuilding – would become particularly knowledgeable about anaerobic exercise, nutrition, supplementation and pharmaceuticals. Bodybuilders making such suggestions recognise these proposals may be discredited by most clinicians but argue that a dismissive attitude is contradictory given medicine's provision of cosmetic surgery and slimming drugs for body beautification. Here bodybuilders claim that with specialist medical assistance the effectiveness of bodybuilding regimes could be maximised and potentially dangerous practices could be more carefully planned, controlled and monitored.

Scientific efforts to limit harm require resources. However, expenditure on research, health and medical treatment is less likely to be forthcoming if disease and illness are caused by 'reprehensible' behaviour (Douglas and Calvez 1990: 463). Also, potential safety benefits may get consumed by performance benefits (Adams 1995). Similar to information acquisition in HIV prevention, knowledge and the establishment of 'trust' may simply lead to increased rather than reduced risk-taking (Scott and Freeman 1995: 162). In making policy recommendations, therefore, tertiary healthcare provision for steroid users would largely or solely be funded by people who live their lives wanting/accepting some non-zero level of risk and who are already willing to invest considerable amounts of time, money and effort into their bodybuilding.

Final word

Recently I attended a university seminar on the nature of 'expertise' and talked with two medical sociologists about bodybuilding, drugs and risk. Their views are typical: 'steroids are dangerous', 'bodybuilders, they're barmy, if they possess any form of expertise, it's not worth knowing about'. These sentiments illustrate Aoki's (1996: 59) point that academics, 'usually circumspect about not denigrating minorities of any type [...] nonetheless too often sneer at bodybuilders'. 'Irrational' risk behaviours such as steroid 'abuse' only confirm widespread suspicion that bodybuilding is a 'shadowy' subculture. Mainstream reactions to drug assisted bodybuilding are comparable to reactions evoked by televised operations of 'disfiguring' cosmetic surgery on the performance artist Orlan: 'indignation that this could be calling itself art; offence at the misuse of medical science [...]; confusion at the apparent pointlessness of the whole exercise' (Goodall 1999: 160).

For good or ill, bodybuilding is an increasingly popular pursuit in the affluent developed world. The 'sport' and 'art' of bodybuilding may arouse indignation, offence and puzzlement among observers but it embodies the resurgence of interest in body modification in the West over the past thirty years (Featherstone 1999). Bodybuilding is one embodied (sub)culturally regulated practice which has gained added momentum following the proliferation of bodily regimens in late modernity. It is neither idiosyncratic nor socially peculiar, and bodybuilders injecting steroids cannot be adequately characterised as 'isolates' (or fatalists) with low group integration. Contemporary bodybuilding is illustrative of many people's increasing desire and tendency to assert control and ownership over the 'natural' object of the human body, to technologically refashion the body according to (sub)cultural designs and emergent dispositions.

Following theoretical arguments that we inhabit a 'risk society' (Beck 1992), bodybuilding illustrates the potential dangers and benefits of technological body modification. It also suggests medical authority may have been weakening as traditional sources of expertise are increasingly being challenged (Gabe *et al.* 1994). Although clinicians have warned bodybuilders and other athletes about steroid risks, many gym members reject these warnings by using various drugs to create and maintain types of muscular body. Such risk behaviour, as demonstrated, is the product of preference rather than a weakness of understanding. Potentially serious health risks attendant to steroid abuse are acknowledged by bodybuilders and efforts are made to manage drug side effects. However, while practising ethnopharmacologists often rely upon subcultural knowledge, there is a pluralism of expertise: clinician's warnings may be rejected but a sense of uncertainty renders many bodybuilders receptive to medicine's role as a potential source of knowledge and practical help. Tertiary healthcare provision remains a possibility for steroid users in general and drug-using bodybuilders in particular. An ethnography of bodybuilding, drugs and risk – in rendering 'fatal' and 'atavistic' behaviour intelligible and reasonable – empirically grounds social scientific debate about the body and self-identity *and* provides necessary data for health interventions aimed at risk reduction. Bodybuilding, a technological form of embodiment, highlights the importance of bringing 'lived bodies' back into social theory and medical practice.

Bibliography

Adams, J. (1995) *Risk*, London: UCL Press.

Adler, P.A. and Adler, P. (1987) *Membership Roles in Field Research*, London: Sage.

American Academy of Pediatrics (1997) 'Adolescents and anabolic steroids: a subject review', *Pediatrics* 99, 6: 904–8.

Annandale, E. (1998) *The Sociology of Health & Medicine: a Critical Introduction*, Oxford: Blackwell.

Aoki, D. (1996) 'Sex and muscle: the female bodybuilder meets Lacan', *Body & Society* 2, 4: 59–74.

Augé, W. and Augé, S. (1999) 'Naturalistic observation of athletic drug-use patterns and behavior in professional-caliber bodybuilders', *Substance Use & Misuse* 34, 2: 217–49.

Balsamo, A. (1996) *Technologies of the Gendered Body*, London: Duke University Press.

— (1995) 'Forms of technological embodiment: reading the body in contemporary culture', *Body & Society* 1, 3–4: 215–37.

Beck, U. (1992) *Risk Society: Towards a New Modernity*, London: Sage.

Becker, H. (1967) 'History, culture and subjective experience', *The Journal of Health and Social Behaviour* 8: 163–76.

— (1963) *Outsiders: Studies in the Sociology of Deviance*. New York: Free Press.

Bednarek, J. (1985) 'Pumping iron or pulling strings: different ways of working out and getting involved in body-building', *International Review for the Sociology of Sport* 20, 4: 239–58.

Bellaby, P. (1990) 'To risk or not to risk? Uses and limitations of Mary Douglas on risk-acceptability for understanding health and safety at work and road accidents', *Sociological Review* 38: 465–83.

Berger, P. and Luckman, T. (1966) *The Social Construction of Reality: A Treatise in the Sociology of Knowledge*, New York: Doubleday & Company, Inc.

Bhasin, S., Storer, T., Berman, N., Callegari, C., Clevenger, B., Phillips, J., Bunnell, T., Tricker, R., Shirazi, A. and Casaburi, R. (1996) 'The effects of supraphysiologic doses of testosterone on muscle size and strength in normal men', *New England Journal of Medicine* 335, 1: 1–7.

Bittner, E. (1965) 'The concept of organisation', reprinted in R. Turner (ed.) (1974) *Ethnomethodology*, Middlesex: Penguin.

Bjorkqvist, K., Nygren, T., Bjorklund, A. and Bjorkqvist, S. (1994) 'Testosterone intake and aggressiveness: real effect or anticipation?' *Aggressive Behaviour* 20, 1: 17–26.

Blake, A. (1996) *The Body Language: the Meaning of Modern Sport*, London: Lawrence & Wishart.

Bloor, M. (1995) *The Sociology of HIV Transmission*, London: Sage.

—— (1978) 'On the analysis of observational data: a discussion of the worth and uses of inductive techniques and respondent validation', *Sociology* 12: 542–52.

Bloor, M., Monaghan, L., Dobash, R.P and Dobash R.E. (1998) 'The body as a chemistry experiment: steroid use among South Wales bodybuilders', in S. Nettleton and J. Watson (eds) *The Body in Everyday Life*, London: Routledge.

Blumer, H.(1969) *Symbolic Interactionism: Perspective and Method*, New Jersey: Prentice Hall.

Bolin, A. (1992a) 'Vandalized vanity: feminine physiques betrayed and portrayed', in F. Mascia-Lees and P. Sharpe (eds) *Tattoo, Torture, Mutilation, and Adornment: The Denaturalization of the Body in Culture and Text*, Albany, NY: State University of New York Press.

Bolin, A. (1992b) 'Flex appeal, food, and fat: competitive bodybuilding, gender, and diet', *Play and Culture* 5: 378–400.

Bordo, S. (1993) *Unbearable Weight: Feminism, Western Culture and the Body*, Berkeley: University of California Press.

Borre, K. (1991) 'Seal blood, Inuit blood, and diet: a biocultural model of physiology and cultural identity', *Medical Anthropology Quarterly* 5, 1: 48–62.

Bourdieu, P. (1992) *The Logic of Practice*, Cambridge: Polity.

—— (1986) 'The forms of capital', in J. Richardson (ed.) *Handbook of Theory and Research for the Sociology of Education*, New York: Greenwood Press.

Bourdieu, P., Darbel, A. and Schnapper, D. (1991) *The Love of Art: European Art Museums and their Public*, Oxford: Polity.

Brain, R. (1979) *The Decorated Body*, New York: Harper and Row.

Brainum, J. (1996) 'Drug world', *Joe Weider's Flex*, June: 165–8.

Brake, M. (1980) *The Sociology of Youth Culture and Youth Subcultures: Sex and Drugs and Rock 'n' Roll?* London: Routledge.

Britton, C. (1998) '"Feeling letdown": an exploration of an embodied sensation associated with breastfeeding', in S. Nettleton and J. Watson (eds) *The Body in Everyday Life*, London: Routledge.

Bromley, R. (1997) 'Review article. The body language: the meaning of modern sport', *Body & Society* 3,1: 1–7.

Brower, K., Blow, F. and Hill, E. (1994) 'Risk factors for anabolic steroid use in men', *Journal of Psychiatric Research* 28, 4: 369–80.

Brower, K., Blow, F., Young, J. and Hill, E. (1991) 'Symptoms and correlates of anabolic-androgenic steroid dependence', *British Journal of Addiction* 86: 759–68.

Burgess, R. (1993) 'Pumping iron or drugs?' in H. Shapiro (ed.) *The Steroid Papers*, London: Institute for the Study of Drug Dependence.

Carter, S. (1995) 'Boundaries of danger and uncertainty: an analysis of the technological culture of risk assessment', in J. Gabe (ed.) *Medicine, Health and Risk: Sociological Approaches*, Oxford: Blackwell.

Cashmore (1998) 'Between mind and muscle', *Body & Society* 4, 2: 83–90.

Choi, P. and Pope, H. (1994) 'Violence toward women and illicit androgenic-anabolic steroid use', *Annals of Clinical Psychiatry* 6, 1: 21–5.

Choi, P., Parrott, A. and Cowan, D. (1989) 'Adverse behavioural effects of anabolic steroids in athletes: a brief review', *Clinical Sports Medicine* 1: 183–7.

Coffey, A. and Atkinson, P. (1996) *Making Sense of Qualitative Data: Complementary Research Strategies*, London: Sage.

Cohen, S. (1980) *Folk Devils and Moral Panics: The Creation of the Mods and Rockers*, Oxford: Martin Robertson.

Collins, H. and Pinch (1998) *The Golem at Large: What You Should Know About Technology*, Cambridge: Cambridge University Press

Connell, R. (1995) *Masculinities*, Cambridge: Polity.

— (1987) *Gender and Power*, Cambridge: Polity.

Cooke, P. (1987) 'Wales', in P. Damesick and P. Wood (eds) *Regional Problems, Problem Regions and Public Policy in the UK*, Oxford: Oxford University Press.

Cooley, C. (1983) *Human Nature and Social Order*, London: Transaction. (Orig. 1902)

Crossley, N. (1996) 'Body-subject/body-power: agency, inscription and control in Foucault and Merleau-Ponty', *Body & Society* 2, 2: 99–116.

— (1995) 'Merleau-Ponty, the elusive body and carnal sociology', *Body & Society* 1, 1: 43–63.

Davis, F. and Munoz, L. (1968) 'Heads and freaks: patterns and meanings of drug use among hippies', *Journal of Health and Social Behaviour* 9: 156–64.

Day, G. (1990) 'Pose for thought: bodybuilding and other matters', in G. Day (ed.) *Readings in Popular Culture: Trivial Pursuits*, New York: St. Martins Press.

Douglas, M. (1990) 'Risk as a forensic resource', *Daedalus* 119: 1–16.

— (1985) *Risk Acceptability according to the Social Sciences*, New York: Russell Sage Foundation.

— (1966) *Purity and Danger: An Analysis of the Concepts of Pollution and Taboo*, London: Routledge.

Douglas, M. and Calvez, M. (1990) 'The self as risk taker: a cultural theory of contagion in relation to AIDS', *Sociological Review* 38: 445–64.

Douglas, M. and Wildavsky, A. (1982) *Risk and Culture: An Essay on the Selection of Technical and Environmental Dangers*, Berkeley: University of California Press.

Duchaine, D. (1989) *Underground Steroid Handbook II*, USA: Daniel Duchaine.

Durkheim, E. (1964) *Rules of Sociological Method*, New York: Free Press. (Orig. 1895)

Edwards, D. and Potter, J. (1992) *Discursive Psychology*, London: Sage.

Elias, N. (1978) *The Civilizing Process*, New York: Urizen.

BIBLIOGRAPHY

Epstein, S. (1996) *Impure Science: Aids, Activism, and the Politics of Knowledge*, London: University of California Press.

Etkin, N. (1993) 'Anthropological methods in ethnopharmacology', *Journal of Ethnopharmacology* 38: 93–104.

Evans, N. (1997) 'Gym and tonic: a profile of 100 male steroid users', *British Journal of Sports Medicine* 31, 1: 54–8.

Falk, P. (1995) 'Written in the flesh', *Body & Society* 1, 1: 95–105.

Faludi, S. (1999) *Stiffed: The Betrayal of the Modern Man*, London: Chatto & Windus.

Featherstone, M. (1999) 'Body modification: an introduction', *Body & Society* 5, 2–3: 1–13.

—— (1992) 'The heroic life and everyday life', *Theory, Culture & Society* 9: 159–82.

—— (1991) 'The body in consumer culture', in M. Featherstone, M. Hepworth, and B. Turner (eds) *The Body: Social Process and Cultural Theory*, London: Sage.

Fieldhouse, P. (1995) *Food and Nutrition: Customs and Culture* (2nd edition), London: Chapman & Hall.

Foucault, M. (1988) 'The dangerous individual', in L. Kritzman (ed.) *Michel Foucault: Politics, Philosophy, Culture: Interviews and Other Writings 1977–1984*, New York: Routledge.

—— (1986) *The Care of the Self: Volume Three of the History of Sexuality*, New York: Pantheon Books.

—— (1983) 'The subject and power', in H. Dreyfus and P. Rabinow, *Michel Foucault: Beyond Structuralism and Hermeneutics* (2nd edition), Chicago: University of Chicago Press.

—— (1980) 'Body-power', in C. Gordon (ed.) *Power/Knowledge*, Brighton: Harvester.

—— (1979) *Discipline and Punish: The Birth of the Prison*, Harmondsworth: Penguin.

—— (1973) *The Birth of the Clinic: An Archaeology of Medical Perception*, London: Tavistock.

Fountain, J., Griffiths, P., Farrell, M., Gossop, M. and Strong, J. (1996) *A Qualitative Study of Patterns of Prescription Drug Use Amongst Chronic Drug Users*, Report to the Department of Health for England, Scotland and Wales.

Fox, N. (1998) '"Risks", "hazards" and life choices: reflections on health at work', *Sociology* 32, 4: 665–87.

Frake, C. (1980) 'The diagnosis of disease among the Subanun of Mindanao', *Language and Cultural Description: Essays by Charles O. Frake*, California: Stanford University Press.

Francis, B. and Reynolds, W. (1989) *Bev Francis' Power Bodybuilding*, New York: Sterling Publishing.

Frank, A. (1997) 'Blurred inscriptions of health and illness', *Body & Society* 3, 2: 103–13.

—— (1995) 'Review symposium: as much as theory can say about bodies', *Body & Society* 1, 1: 184–7.

—— (1991) 'For a sociology of the body: an analytic review', in M. Featherstone, M. Hepworth, and B. Turner (eds) *The Body: Social Process and Cultural Theory*, London: Sage.

—— (1990) 'Bringing bodies back in: a decade review', *Theory, Culture and Society* 7, 1: 131–62.

BIBLIOGRAPHY

Friedl, K. and Yesalis, C. (1989) 'Self-treatment of gynecomastia in bodybuilders who use anabolic steroids', *The Physician and Sportsmedicine* 17: 67– 79.

Fussell, S. (1994) 'Bodybuilder Americanus', in L. Goldstein (ed.) *The Male Body: Features, Destinies, Exposures*, Michigan: University of Michigan Press.

— (1991) *Muscle: Confessions of an Unlikely Bodybuilder*, New York: Avon Books.

Gabe, J., Kelleher, D. and Williams, G. (eds) (1994) *Challenging Medicine*, London: Routledge.

Gaines, C. and Butler, G. (1974) *Pumping Iron: The Art and Sport of Bodybuilding*, New York: Simon and Schuster.

Garfinkel, H. (1967) *Studies in Ethnomethodology*, New York: Prentice-Hall.

Gatens, M. (1996) *Imaginary Bodies: Ethics, Power and Corporeality*, London: Routledge.

Giddens, A. (1991) *Modernity and Self-Identity: Self and Society in the Late Modern Age*, Cambridge: Polity Press.

Gilbert, B. (1993) 'Introduction', in C. Yesalis (ed.) *Anabolic Steroids in Sport and Exercise*, Leeds: Human Kinetics.

Gillett, J. and White, P. (1992) 'Male bodybuilding and the reassertion of hegemonic masculinity: a critical feminist perspective', *Play and Culture* 5: 358–69.

Glaser, B. and Strauss, A. (1967) *The Discovery of Grounded Theory*, Chicago: Aldine.

Glassner, B. (1990) 'Fit for postmodern selfhood', in H. Becker and M. McCall (eds) *Symbolic Interaction and Cultural Studies*, Chicago: University of Chicago Press.

Goffman, E. (1989) 'On fieldwork', *Journal of Contemporary Ethnography* 18, 2: 123–32.

— (1968) *Stigma: Notes on the Management of Spoiled Identity*, Middlesex: Penguin Books.

— (1963) *Behavior in Public Places: Notes on the Social Organization of Gatherings*, New York: Free Press.

— (1961) *Asylums: Essays on the Social Situation of Mental Patients and Other Inmates*, New York: Anchor Books.

Goldstein, P. (1990) 'Anabolic steroids: an ethnographic approach', in G. Lin and L. Erinoff (eds) *Anabolic Steroid Abuse*, Rockville, MD: US Dept. of Health and Human Services.

Goldstein, P. and Lee, K. (1994) 'Anabolic-androgenic steroid use and violence: a preliminary analysis', Paper presented to *The American Public Health Association*, Washington DC.

Goodall, J. (1999) 'An order of pure decision: un-natural selection in the work of Stelarc and Orlan', *Body & Society* 5, 2–3: 149–70.

Green, J. (1997a) 'Risk and the construction of social identity: children's talk about accidents', *Sociology of Health & Illness* 19, 4: 457–79.

— (1997b) *Risk and Misfortune: The Social Construction of Accidents*, London: UCL Press.

Grivetti, L. and Pangborn, R. (1974) 'Origin of selected old testament dietary prohibitions', *Journal of American Dietetic Association* 65: 634–8.

Grunding, P. and Bachmann, M. (1995) *World Anabolic Review 1996*, M.B. Muscle Books.

Guthrie, S. and Catelnuovo, S. (1992) 'Elite women bodybuilders: models of resistance or compliance?' *Play and Culture* 5: 401–8.

Hamilton, C. and Collins, J. (1981) 'The role of alcohol in wife beating and child abuse', in J. Collins (ed.) *Drinking and Crime*, London: Tavistock.

Hammersley, M. (1992) *What's Wrong With Ethnography?* London: Routledge.

BIBLIOGRAPHY

Hammersley, M. and Atkinson, P. (1995) *Ethnography: Principles in Practice* (2nd edition), London: Routledge.

Hargreaves, J. (1997) 'Women's boxing and related activities: introducing images and meanings', *Body & Society* 3, 4: 33–49.

Harris, C. (1987) *Redundancy and Recession in South Wales*, Oxford: Blackwells.

Hart, G. and Flowers, P. (1996) 'Recent developments in the sociology of HIV risk behaviour', *Risk Decision and Policy* 1, 2: 153–65.

Hart, M. (undated) 'Nubaine: all pain. No gain', *Mick Hart's No Bull Collection* 10: 12–15.

Hebdige, D. (1979) *Subculture: The Meaning of Style*, London: Routledge.

Hesse, M. (1980) *Revolutions and Reconstructions in the Philosophy of Science*, Brighton: Harvester Wheatsheaf.

Holstein, J. and Gubrium, J. (1997) 'Active interviewing', in D. Silverman (ed.) *Qualitative Research: Theory, Method and Practice*, London: Sage.

Hunt, J. (1995) 'Divers' accounts of normal risk', *Symbolic Interaction* 18, 4: 439–62.

Jackson, S. (1996) 'Heterosexuality as a problem for feminist theory', in L. Adkins and V. Merchant (eds) *Sexualising the Social: Power and the Organization of Sexuality*, London: Macmillan.

Jefferson, T. (1998) 'Muscle, hard men and Iron Mike Tyson: reflections on desire, anxiety and the embodiment of masculinity', *Body & Society* 4, 1: 77–98.

Kane, P. (1994) 'New men in the making', *The Guardian* 12th September.

Kashkin, K. (1992) 'Anabolic steroids', in L. Lowinsohn, P. Ruiz, R. Millman and J. Langrid (eds) *Substance Abuse: A Comprehensive Textbook*, Baltimore: Williams and Wilkins.

Kennedy, R. (1983) *Hard-Core Bodybuilding: the Blood, Sweat and Tears of Pumping Iron*. New York: Sterling

Kimmel, M. (1994) 'Consuming manhood: the feminization of American culture and the recreation of the male body, 1832–1920', in L. Goldstein (ed.) *The Male Body: Features, Destinies, Exposures*, Michigan: University of Michigan Press.

Klein, A. (1995) 'Life's too short to die small: steroid use among male bodybuilders', in D. Sabo and F. Gordon (eds) *Men's Health and Illness: Gender, Power, and the Body*, London: Sage.

—— (1993) *Little Big Men: Bodybuilding Subculture and Gender Construction*, Albany, NY: State University of New York Press.

—— (1992) 'Man makes himself: alienation and self-objectification in bodybuilding', *Play and Culture* 5: 326–37.

—— (1986) 'Pumping Irony: Crisis and Contradiction in Bodybuilding', *Sociology of Sport Journal* 3: 112–33.

Klesse, C. (1999) '"Modern primitivism": non-mainstream body modification and racialized representation', *Body & Society* 5, 2–3, 15–38.

Kochakian, C. (1993) 'Anabolic-androgenic steroids: a historical perspective and definition', in C. Yesalis (ed.) *Anabolic Steroids in Sports and Exercise*, Leeds: Human Kinetics.

Korkia, P. and Stimson, G. (1993) *Anabolic Steroid Use In Great Britain: An Exploratory Investigation*, London: The Centre for Research on Drugs and Health Behaviour.

BIBLIOGRAPHY

Lane, K. (1995) 'The medical model of the body as a site of risk: a case study of childbirth', in J. Gabe (ed.) *Medicine, Health and Risk: Sociological Approaches*, Oxford: Blackwell.

Lasch, C. (1980) *The Culture of Narcissism: American Life in an Age of Diminishing Expectations*, London: Abacus.

Leder, D. (1990) *The Absent Body*, Chicago: University of Chicago Press.

Lenehan, P., Bellis, M. and McVeigh, J. (1996) 'A study of anabolic steroid use in the North West of England', *The Journal of Performance Enhancing Drugs* 1, 57–70.

Lowe, M. (1998) *Women of Steel: Female Bodybuilders and the Struggle for Self-Definition*, New York: New York University Press.

Lubell, A. (1989) 'Does steroid abuse cause – or excuse – violence?' *The Physician and Sportsmedicine* 17: 176–85.

Lupton, D. (1997) *The Imperative of Health: Public Health and the Regulated Body*, London: Sage.

Lupton and Tulloch (1998) 'The adolescent "unfinished body", reflexivity and HIV/AIDS risk', *Body & Society* 4, 2: 19–34.

Macandrew, C. and Edgerton, R. (1970) *Drunken Comportment: A Social Explanation*, London: Nelson.

McArdle, W., Fank, K. and Katch, V. (1986) *Exercise Physiology: Energy, Nutrition and Human Performance* (2nd edition), Philadelphia: Lea & Febiger.

McBride, A., Petersen, T. and Williamson, K. (1998) 'Working with androgenic anabolic steroid users', in M. Bloor and F. Wood (eds) *Addictions and Problem Drug Use: Issues in Behaviour, Policy and Practice*. London: Jessica Kingsley.

McBride, A., Williamson, K. and Peterson, T. (1996) 'Three cases of Nalbuphine Hydro-chloride dependence associated with anabolic steroid use', *British Journal of Sports Medicine* 9: 13–24.

McDonald-Walker (1998) 'Fighting the legacy: British Bikers in the 1990s', *Sociology* 32, 2: 379–96.

McKeganey, N. (1990) 'Drug abuse in the community: needle-sharing and the risk of HIV infection', in S. Cunningham-Burley and N. McKeganey (eds) *Readings in Medical Sociology*, London: Routledge.

McKeganey N. and Barnard, M. (1992) *Aids, Drugs and Sexual Risk: Lives in the Balance*, Buckingham: Open University Press.

McKeown, T. (1979) *The Role of Medicine: Dream, Mirage or Nemesis*, (2nd ed.) Oxford: Blackwell Scientific.

McKillop, G. (1987) 'Drug abuse in bodybuilders in the West of Scotland', *Scottish Medical Journal* 32: 39–41.

Manning, K. and Fabrega, H. (1973) 'The experience of self and body: health and illness in the Chiapas Highlands', in G. Psathas (ed.) *Phenomenological Sociology*, London: Wiley & Sons.

Mansfield, A. and McGinn, B. (1993) 'Pumping irony: the muscular and the feminine', in S. Scott and D. Morgan (eds) *Body Matters*, London: Falmer Press.

Matza, D. (1969) *Becoming Deviant*, New Jersey: Prentice-Hall.

Mauss, M. (1973) 'Techniques of the body', *Economy and Society* 2, 1: 70–88. (Orig. 1934)

BIBLIOGRAPHY

Mead, G.H. (1934) *Mind, Self and Society*, Chicago: University of Chicago Press.

Mellor, P. and Shilling, C. (1997) *Re-forming the Body: Religion, Community and Modernity*, London: Sage.

Mennell, S., Murcott, A. and Van Otterloo, A. (1992) *The Sociology of Food: Eating, Diet and Culture*, London: Sage.

Merleau-Ponty, M. (1962) *The Phenomenology of Perception*, London: Routledge.

Messner, M. and Sabo, D. (1994) *Sex, Violence & Power in Sports: Rethinking Masculinity*, California: The Crossing Press.

Millar, A. (1994) 'Licit steroid use – hope for the future', *British Journal of Sports Medicine* 28, 2: 79–83.

Miller, J. and Glassner, B. (1997) 'The "inside" and the "outside": finding realities in interviews', in D. Silverman (ed.) *Qualitative Research: Theory, Method and Practice*, London: Sage.

Monaghan, L. (2001) 'The bodybuilding ethnophysiology thesis', in N. Watson (ed.) *Re-framing the Body*, London: Macmillan.

— (1999a) 'Accessing a demonised subculture: studying drug use and violence among bodybuilders', in L. Noakes, E. Wincup and F. Brookman (eds) *Qualitative Research In Criminology*, Aldershot: Ashgate

— (1999b) 'Challenging medicine? Bodybuilding, drugs and risk', *Sociology of Health & Illness* 21, 6: 707–34.

Monaghan, L., Bloor, M., Dobash, R.P. and Dobash, R.E. (1998) 'Bodybuilding and sexual attractiveness', in J. Richardson and A. Shaw (eds) *The Body in Qualitative Research*, Aldershot: Ashgate.

Moore, D. (1993) 'Social controls, harm minimisation and interactive outreach: the public health implications of an ethnography of drug use', *Australian Journal of Public Health* 17, 1: 58–67.

Morgan, D. (1993) 'You too can have a body like mine: reflections on the male body and masculinities', in S. Scott and D. Morgan (eds) *Body Matters*, London: Falmer Press.

Moss, D. (1988) 'And now the steroid defence?' *American Bar Association Journal* 1: 22–4.

Mullen, K. (1990) 'Drink is all right in moderation: accounts of alcohol use and abuse from male Glaswegians', in S. Cunningham-Burley and N. McKeganey (eds) *Readings in Medical Sociology*, London: Routledge.

Nazroo, J. (1997) *The Health of Britain's Ethnic Minorities*, London: Policy Studies Institute.

Nettleton, S. (1995) *The Sociology of Health and Illness*, Cambridge: Polity Press.

Nettleton, S. and Watson, J. (eds) (1998) *The Body in Everyday Life*, London: Routledge.

Pates, R. and Barry, C. (1996) 'Steroid use in Cardiff: a problem for whom?' Paper presented to *The 7th International Conference on the Reduction of Drug Related Harm*, Hobart, Tasmania.

Pates, R. and Temple, D. (1992) *The Use of Anabolic Steroids in Wales: A Report by the Welsh Committee on Drug Misuse*, Cardiff: Welsh Office.

Phillips, B. (1997a) 'Uncensored Q & A', *Muscle-Media 2000* March: 38–46.

— (1997b) 'No holds barred', *Muscle-Media 2000* February: 10–13.

BIBLIOGRAPHY

— (1997c) 'Letters: readers' feedback', *Muscle-Media 2000* March: 20–1.

— (1996) 'No holds barred', *Muscle-Media 2000* September: 10–13.

Phillips, W. (1991) *Anabolic Reference Guide* (6th Issue), USA: Mile High Publishing.

Pitts, V. (1998) '"Reclaiming" the female body: embodied identity work, resistance, and the grotesque', *Body & Society* 4, 3: 67–84.

Polhemus, T. (1978) *Social Aspects of the Human Body*, Middlesex: Penguin Books.

Pope, H., Gruber, A., Choi, P., Olivardia, R. and Phillips, K. (1997) 'Muscle dysmorphia: an underrecognized form of body dysmorphic disorder', *Psychosomatics* 38: 548–57.

Pope, H. and Katz, D. (1990) 'Homicide and near homicide by anabolic steroid users', *Journal of Clinical Psychiatry* 51, 1: 28–31.

Rhodes, T. (1997) 'Risk theory in epidemic times: sex, drugs and the social organisation of "risk behaviour"', *Sociology of Health & Illness* 19, 2: 208–27.

Rhodes, T. and Stimson, G. (1998) 'Community intervention among hidden populations of injecting drug users in the time of AIDS', in M. Bloor and F. Wood (eds) *Addictions and Problem Drug Use: Issues in Behaviour, Policy and Practice*, London: Jessica Kingsley.

Riem, K. and Hursey, K. (1995) 'Using anabolic-androgenic steroids to enhance physique and performance: effects on mood and behaviour', *Clinical Psychological Review* 15, 3: 235–56.

Robillard, A. (1999) 'Wild phenomena and disability jokes', *Body & Society* 5, 4: 61–5.

Sabo, D. and Gordon, F. (eds) (1995) *Men's Health and Illness: Gender, Power, and the Body*, London: Sage.

Sabo, D. and Jansen, S. (1994) 'Seen but not heard: images of black men in sports media', in M. Messner and D. Sabo (1994) *Sex, Violence & Power in Sports: Rethinking Masculinity*, California: The Crossing Press.

Salisbury, J. (1994) 'Becoming Qualified: An Ethnography of a Post Experience Teacher Training Course', Unpublished PhD thesis, University of Wales, College of Cardiff.

Sartre, J. (1958) *Being and Nothingness*, London: Methuan and Co.

Schulze, L. (1990) 'On the muscle', in J. Gaines and C. Herzog (eds) *Fabrications: Costume and the Female Body*, London: Routledge.

Schutz, A. (1970) *Reflections on the Problem of Relevance*, New Haven: Yale University Press.

— (1967) *Collected Papers I: The Problem of Social Reality*, The Hague: Martinus Nijhoff.

— (1964) *Collected Papers II: Studies in Social Theory*, The Hague: Martinus Nijhoff.

Scott, M. and Lyman, S. (1968) 'Accounts', *American Sociological Review* 33: 46–62.

Scott, S. and Freeman, R. (1995) 'Prevention as a problem of modernity: the example of HIV and AIDS', in J. Gabe (ed.) *Medicine, Health and Risk: Sociological Approaches*, Oxford: Blackwell.

Scott, S., Jackson, S. and Backett-Milburn, K. (1998) 'Swings and roundabouts: risk anxiety and the everyday worlds of children', *Sociology* 32, 4: 689–705.

Seidel, J. and Clark, J. (1984) 'The ethnograph: a computer program for the analysis of qualitative data', *Qualitative Sociology* 7: 110–25.

Shildrick (1998) 'Book review. Deviant bodies: critical perspectives on science and difference in popular culture', *Body & Society* 4, 1: 113–15.

BIBLIOGRAPHY

Shilling, C. (1993) *The Body and Social Theory*, London: Sage.

Shilling, C. and Mellor, P. (1996) 'Embodiment, structuration theory and modernity: mind/body dualism and the repression of sensuality', *Body & Society* 2, 4:1–15.

Silverman, D. (1993) *Interpreting Qualitative Data: Methods for Analysing Talk, Text and Interaction*, London: Sage.

Smith, G. (1997) 'Incivil attention and everyday intolerance: vicissitudes of exercising in public places', *Perspectives on Social Problems* 9: 59–79.

Spradley, J. (1979) *The Ethnographic Interview*, New York: Holt, Rinehart and Winston.

Stewart-Clevidence, B. and Goldstein, P. (1996) 'A female ethnographer in a macho milieu: doing research on anabolic androgenic steroids', *The Journal of Performance Enhancing Drugs* 1, 1: 33–40.

St Martin, L. and Gavey, N. (1996) 'Women's bodybuilding: feminist resistance and/or femininity's recuperation?' *Body & Society* 2, 4: 45–57.

Strauss, R. and Yesalis, C. (1993) 'Additional effects of anabolic steroids on women', in C. Yesalis (ed.) *Anabolic Steroids in Sports and Exercise*, Leeds: Human Kinetics.

Street, C., Antonio, J. and Cudlipp, D. (1996) 'Androgen use by athletes: a re-evaluation of the health risks', *Canadian Journal of Applied Physiology* 21, 6: 421–40.

Sweetman, P. (1999) 'Anchoring the (postmodern) self? Body modification, fashion and identity', *Body & Society* 5, 2–3: 51–76.

Sykes, G. and Matza, D. (1957) 'Techniques of neutralization: a theory of delinquency', *American Sociological Review* 22: 664–70.

Taylor, A. (1993) *Women Drug Users: An Ethnography of a Female Injecting Community*, Oxford: Clarendon Press.

Taylor, I., Walton, P. and Young, J. (1973) *The New Criminology: for a Social Theory of Deviance*, London: Routledge.

Thirer, J. and Greer, D. (1978) 'Competitive bodybuilding: sport, art or exhibitionism?' *Journal of Sport Behaviour* 1, 4: 186–94.

Todd, T. (1987) 'Anabolic steroids: the gremlins of sport', *Journal of Sport History* 14, 1: 87–107.

Turner, B. (1999) 'The possibility of primitiveness: towards a sociology of body marks in cool societies', *Body & Society* 5, 2–3: 39–50.

— (1996) *The Body and Society* (2nd edition), London: Sage.

— (1992) *Regulating Bodies: Essays in Medical Sociology*, London: Routledge.

— (1991a) 'Recent developments in the theory of the body', in M. Featherstone, M. Hepworth, and B. Turner (eds) *The Body: Social Process and Cultural Theory*, London: Sage.

— (1991b) 'The discourse of diet', in M. Featherstone, M. Hepworth, and B. Turner (eds) *The Body: Social Process and Cultural Theory*, London: Sage.

Uzych, L. (1992) 'Anabolic androgenic steroids and psychiatric related effects: a review', *Canadian Journal of Psychiatry Review* 37, 1: 23–8.

Wachter, F. (1984) 'The symbolism of the healthy body: a philosophical analysis of the sportive imagery of health', *Journal of the Philosophy of Sport* XI: 56–62.

BIBLIOGRAPHY

Wacquant, L. (1995a) 'Pugs at work: bodily capital and bodily labour among professional boxers', *Body & Society* 1, 1: 65–93.

— (1995b) 'Review article: why men desire muscles', *Body & Society*, 1, 1: 163–79.

Watson, J. (2000) *Male Bodies: Health, Culture and Identity*, Buckingham: OUP.

— (1998) 'Running around like a lunatic', in S. Nettleton and J. Watson (eds) *The Body in Everyday Life*, London: Routledge.

Watson, J., Cunningham Burley, S. and Watson, N. (1995) 'Lay theorising about the body and health', paper presented to the *British Sociological Association Medical Sociology Group 27th Annual Conference*, University of York, 22–24 September.

Weber, C. (1996) 'Never say never: Dennis Newman talks about his long road to recovery', *Muscular Development* May: 136–38, 188.

Weber, M. (1976) *The Protestant Ethic and the Spirit of Capitalism*, London: Allen and Unwin. (Orig. 1905)

Weinstein, R. (1980) 'Vocabularies of motive for illicit drug use: an application of the accounts framework', *The Sociological Quarterly* 21: 577–93.

White, P. and Gillett, J. (1994) 'Reading the muscular body: a critical decoding of advertisements in *Flex* magazine', *Sociology of Sport Journal* 11: 19–39.

Whitehead, S. (1999) 'Hegemonic masculinity revisited', *Gender, Work and Organization* 6, 1: 58–62.

Widdicombe, S. and Wooffitt, R. (1995) *The Language of Youth Subcultures: Social Identity in Action,* Hertfordshire: Harvester Wheatsheaf.

Wight, D. (1999) 'Cultural factors in young heterosexual men's perception of HIV risk', *Sociology of Health & Illness* 21, 6: 735–58.

Williams, G., Popay, J. and Bissell, P. (1995) 'Public health risks in the material world: barriers to social movements in health', in J. Gabe (ed.) *Medicine, Health and Risk: Sociological Approaches*, Oxford: Blackwell.

Williams, S. and Bendelow, G. (1998) 'Malignant bodies: children's beliefs about health', in S. Nettleton and J. Watson (eds) *The Body in Everyday Life*, London: Routledge.

Williamson, D. (1994) 'The psychological effects of anabolic steroids', *The International Journal of Drug Policy* 5, 1: 18–22.

Williamson, K., Davies, M. and McBride, A. (1993) 'A well steroid user clinic', in H. Shapiro (ed.) *The Steroid Papers*, London: Institute for the Study of Drug Dependence.

Willis, P. (1977) 'The cultural meaning of drug abuse', in S. Hall and J. Jefferson (eds) *Resistance Through Rituals: Youth Subculture in Post-war Britain*, London: Hutchinson University Library.

Wormley, C. and Clarke, C. (1995) *The 1995/1996 U.K Steroid Guide*, Edwards publishing.

Wright, J. (1982) *Anabolic Steroids and Sports: Volume II*, Natick, MA: Sports Science Consultants.

Yates, D. (1994) 'Quote, unquote: Mr Olympia', *For Him Magazine* 92.

Yesalis, C. (ed.) (1993) *Anabolic Steroids in Sports and Exercise*, Leeds: Human Kinetics.

Yesalis, C. (1992) 'Epidemiology and patterns of anabolic-androgenic steroid use', *Psychiatric Annals* 22: 7–18.

BIBLIOGRAPHY

Yesalis, C., Vicary, J., Buckley, W., Streit, A., Katz, D. and Wright, J. (1990) 'Indications of psychological dependence among anabolic-steroid abusers', in G. Lin and L. Erinoff (eds) *Anabolic Steroid Abuse*, Rockville, MD: US Dept. of Health and Human Services.

Young, J. (1972) *The Drug Takers: The Social Meaning of Drug Use*, London: Granada Publishing.

Young, K., McTeer, W. and White, P. (1994) 'Body talk: male athletes reflect on sport, injury, and pain', *Sociology of Sport Journal* 11: 175–94.

Zane, F. (1997) 'Spotlight: Frank Zane. An interview by Kal Yee', *Muscle Media* July: 60–5.

Zinberg, N. (1984) *Drug, Set, and Setting*, New Haven: Yale University Press.

208

Index

INDEX